Hypoparathyroidism

Natalie E. Cusano
Editor

Hypoparathyroidism

A Clinical Casebook

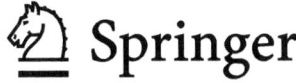 Springer

Editor
Natalie E. Cusano
Department of Medicine
Division of Endocrinology
Northwell Health/Lenox Hill Hospital
New York, NY
USA

ISBN 978-3-030-29432-8   ISBN 978-3-030-29433-5   (eBook)
https://doi.org/10.1007/978-3-030-29433-5

This Springer imprint is published by the registered company Springer Nature Switzerland AG
The registered company address is: Gewerbestrasse 11, 6330 Cham, Switzerland

Preface

The physician's duty is not to stave off death or return patients to their old lives, but to take into our arms a patient and family whose lives have disintegrated and work until they can stand back up and face - and make sense of - their own existence.

– Paul Kalanithi, MD

Hypoparathyroidism is a rare endocrine disease defined by low or insufficient parathyroid hormone concentrations, leading to hypocalcemia and hyperphosphatemia. It has been classified as an orphan disease in the United States and by the European Medicines Agency. Despite being a rare disease, hypoparathyroidism has a profound impact on the lives of affected patients, due in part to the challenge to control serum calcium levels. In addition, chronic manifestations impact quality of life and multiple organs including the renal, neurologic, and skeletal systems. Conventional therapy consists of calcium and active vitamin D supplementation, often in large doses. Hypoparathyroidism was the only classic endocrine deficiency disease for which the replacement hormone was not an approved treatment until 2015, when recombinant human PTH(1–84) [rhPTH(1–84)] was approved for patients with difficult to control disease.

This book is designed to aid in the management of hypoparathyroidism through a patient-focused approach. The authors have provided cases from their extensive background to address some of the challenges in the management of patients with hypoparathyroidism. I would like to acknowledge the authors and patients who have contributed to this field with the expectation that their experiences will help others.

New York, NY, USA   Natalie E. Cusano, MD, MS

Contents

Contributors

Yousef Alalawi, MD McMaster University, Hamilton, ON, Canada

Hajar Abu Alrob, BSc, MSc McMaster University, Hamilton, ON, Canada

Arpita Bhalodkhar, MD Department of Medicine, Division of Endocrinology, Northwell Health/Lenox Hill Hospital, New York, NY, USA

John P. Bilezikian, MD, PhD (honorary) Department of Medicine, Division of Endocrinology, College of Physicians & Surgeons, Columbia University, New York, NY, USA

Bart L. Clarke, MD Mayo Clinic, Rochester, MN, USA

Natalie E. Cusano, MD, MS Department of Medicine, Division of Endocrinology, Northwell Health/Lenox Hill Hospital, New York, NY, USA

Shira B. Eytan, MD Division of Endocrinology, NYU Langone, New York, NY, USA

Rachel I. Gafni, MD Skeletal Disorders and Mineral Homeostasis Section, National Institutes of Dental and Craniofacial Research, National Institutes of Health, Bethesda, MD, USA

Rebecca J. Gordon, MD Division of Endocrinology and Diabetes and the Center for Bone Health, The Children's Hospital of Philadelphia, Philadelphia, PA, USA

Department of Pediatrics, University of Pennsylvania Perelman School of Medicine, Philadelphia, PA, USA

Division of Endocrinology, Boston Children's Hospital, Harvard Medical School, Boston, MA, USA

Steven Ing, MD Division of Endocrinology, Diabetes, & Metabolism, Department of Internal Medicine, Ohio State University Wexner Medical Center, Columbus, OH, USA

Aliya Khan, MD McMaster University, Hamilton, ON, Canada

Michael A. Levine, MD Division of Endocrinology and Diabetes and the Center for Bone Health, The Children's Hospital of Philadelphia, Philadelphia, PA, USA

Department of Pediatrics, University of Pennsylvania Perelman School of Medicine, Philadelphia, PA, USA

E. Pauline Liao, MD Department of Medicine, Division of Endocrinology, Northwell Health/Lenox Hill Hospital, New York, NY, USA

Iman M'Hiri, BSc, MSc Bone Research and Education Centre, Oakville, ON, Canada

Lars Rejnmark, MD, PhD Aarhus University Hospital, Department of Endocrinology and Internal Medicine, Aarhus, Denmark

Kelly L. Roszko, MD, PhD Skeletal Disorders and Mineral Homeostasis Section, National Institutes of Dental and Craniofacial Research, National Institutes of Health, Bethesda, MD, USA

Tanja Sikjaer, MD, PhD Department of Endocrinology and Internal Medicine, Aarhus University Hospital, Aarhus, Denmark

Barbara C. Silva, MD, PhD Division of Endocrinology, Santa Casa Hospital, Belo Horizonte, Brazil

Division of Endocrinology, Felicio Rocho Hospital, Belo Horizonte, Brazil

Department of Medicine, Centro Universitario de Belo Horizonte, UNIBH, Belo Horizonte, Brazil

Melissa Sum, MD Division of Endocrinology, Diabetes and Metabolism, Department of Internal Medicine, New York University School of Medicine, New York, NY, USA

Franco Vallejo, MD Division of Endocrinology, Diabetes and Metabolism, Department of Internal Medicine, New York University School of Medicine, New York, NY, USA

Tamara Vokes, MD Department of Medicine, Section of Endocrinology, University of Chicago, Chicago, IL, USA

Karen K. Winer, MD Eunice Kennedy Shriver National Institute of Child Health and Human Development, NIH, Bethesda, MD, USA

Chapter 1
Acute Postoperative Hypocalcemia After Neck Surgery

Arpita Bhalodkhar and Natalie E. Cusano

Case Presentation

A 49-year-old woman with a history of traumatic left Colles' fracture was referred to endocrine clinic for hypercalcemia of 10.5 mg/dL (normal: 8.6–10.2; albumin 4.5 g/dL) by her orthopedic team. She had no history of nephrolithiasis or prior fractures. Physical exam was grossly unremarkable. Parathyroid sestamibi scan was notable for a focus of increased radiotracer uptake in the right upper thyroid, consistent with a parathyroid adenoma. In addition, there noted to be a second focus of increased uptake in the left lower thyroid which did not persist on delayed imaging and was postulated to represent a thyroid adenoma. Thyroid ultrasound showed a cystic nodule in the

A. Bhalodkhar · N. E. Cusano (✉)
Department of Medicine, Division of Endocrinology,
Northwell Health/Lenox Hill Hospital, New York, NY, USA
e-mail: ncusano@northwell.edu

© Springer Nature Switzerland AG 2020
N. E. Cusano (ed.), *Hypoparathyroidism*,
https://doi.org/10.1007/978-3-030-29433-5_1

right lower lobe and a 2.9 × 1.5 × 2.1 cm heterogeneous, solid, and hypovascular mass. Thyroid fine needle aspiration showed a follicular lesion and could not exclude neoplasm. Repeat laboratory values demonstrated a serum calcium of 11.0 md/dL, PTH 143 pg/mL (normal: 15–65), 25-hydroxyvitamin D 22 mg/dL (normal: 20–80), and a 24-hour urine calcium level of 263 mg (50–250). The plan was for total thyroidectomy and resection of parathyroid adenoma. At the time of surgery, an enlarged posterior right parathyroid adenoma was noted deep in the tracheoesophageal groove, which was dissected and excised. On frozen section, there was the classic parathyroid adenoma appearance. Despite removal of this gland, the patient's intraoperative PTH fell only from 226 pg/mL to 160 pg/mL. Exploration of the left neck revealed a second enlarged parathyroid gland which was resected. The patient's PTH fell to normal levels, and her calcium postoperatively was 9.0 mg/dL. She was discharged on calcium and vitamin D. Pathology was negative for thyroid cancer. Ten days postoperatively, she presented to the thyroid clinic with anxiety, tremor, difficulty concentrating, and insomnia. She was sent to the emergency room for further management. Laboratory values from the emergency department were significant for the following: serum calcium 6.1 mg/dL (albumin 4.3 mg/dL), PTH 11 pg/mL, phosphorus of 8.0 mg/dL (normal: 2.5–4.5), and magnesium 2.1 mg/dL (normal: 1.6–2.6). EKG demonstrated a QTc of 491 msec (normal: ≤440).

Assessment and Diagnosis

This patient had primary hyperparathyroidism with double adenomas and a nodular goiter. She developed acute postoperative hypocalcemia, which can be a true medical emergency. Hypocalcemia is defined as an albumin-adjusted or ionized calcium concentration below the lower limit of the normal range. Serum calcium is corrected for low albumin using the following equation: corrected serum total calcium = measured total calcium + [0.8 × (4.0-measured serum albumin)].

The decision to treat hypocalcemia is determined not only by the calcium level but also by any associated symptoms. The severity of signs and symptoms depends on the absolute calcium level, the rate of decrease in calcium, and individual variability. Some patients with mild hypocalcemia may be highly symptomatic, especially if the serum calcium has dropped acutely. Patients with hypocalcemia that has developed over many years may not have symptoms, despite having a low absolute serum calcium [1].

Approximately 7.6% of anterior neck surgeries result in hypoparathyroidism, of which 75% is transient, defined as lasting less than 6 months. Factors influencing the development of postoperative hypocalcemia include the extent of surgery (greater for total thyroidectomy versus lobectomy), the use of intraoperative PTH measurements for primary hyperparathyroidism (associated with decreased risk), reoperation, and the experience of the surgeon (higher surgical volume decreases risk) [2].

Management

Intravenous calcium administration should be considered for clinical features of hypocalcemia including symptoms of paresthesias, carpopedal spasm, broncho- or laryngospasm, tetany, seizures, mental status changes, positive Chvostek's or Trousseau's signs, bradycardia, impaired cardiac contractility, and prolongation of the QT interval. In addition, although some patients with marked hypocalcemia (i.e., corrected calcium lower than 7.0 mg/dL) may not be symptomatic, intravenous therapy may be indicated because at those levels, life-threatening features such as laryngeal spasm and seizures can appear acutely. Patients who become unable to take or absorb oral supplements can quickly become symptomatic, although the serum calcium may not have fallen dramatically at the time they present with symptoms [1, 3, 4]. Chvostek's sign is elicited by tapping over the facial nerve in front of the tragus, and a positive sign is the twitching of the ipsilateral facial muscles. Of note, approximately 10–25% of healthy individuals will have a positive Chvostek's sign, and it will be negative in 30% of patients with hypocalcemia [5]. Trousseau's sign is elicited by inflating a blood pressure cuff above the systolic blood pressure for 3 minutes, occluding the brachial artery and inducing carpopedal spasm. Trousseau's sign has a sensitivity of 94–99% and is present in only 1% of normocalcemic individuals [6].

The goals of intravenous therapy of hypocalcemia are to control symptoms, reverse signs of hypocalcemia (i.e., prolonged QTc), and restore serum calcium to the lower end of the normal range. This chapter will review dosages for treatment of adults, while the therapy of acute hypocalcemia in children is covered in Chap. 9. The initial dose of intravenous calcium gluconate is 1–2 g (90–180 mg elemental calcium) in 50 mL of 5% dextrose and can be infused over 10–20 minutes. Calcium should not be given more rapidly because of the serious risk of cardiac dysfunction, including systolic arrest. This dose of calcium gluconate typically raises the serum calcium concentration for only several hours. A slower infusion of calcium (10% calcium gluconate, which is 90 mg of elemental calcium per 10 mL) should follow after the acute administration. Since calcium chloride is more likely to cause tissue necrosis if extravasated subcutaneously, calcium gluconate is preferred and can be administered in a peripheral vein. Concentrated calcium solutions are irritating to veins, and thus the calcium should be diluted in dextrose and water or saline. The intravenous solution should not contain bicarbonate or phosphate, however, as both can form insoluble calcium salts. An initial infusion rate would be 50–100 mL/h (equivalent to 50–100 mg/h) and can be adjusted to increase the corrected serum calcium concentration to the lower end of the normal range. This infusion protocol will deliver as much as 15 mg/kg body weight over 8–10 hours and raise the serum calcium levels by approximately 2 mg/dL (0.5 mmol/L). Cardiac monitoring with EKG or telemetry can be considered. Oral calcium should be initiated as soon possible since the effects of intravenous calcium are short. Serum calcium should be monitored very closely, with cessation of the calcium drip once serum calcium has risen and the patient is able to tolerate oral calcium. Calcium carbonate (40% elemental calcium) and calcium citrate (21% elemental calcium) are the most commonly used oral preparations. Calcium carbonate should be taken with meals for best absorption [1, 3, 4].

Active vitamin D metabolites should also be considered, although the onset of action is typically 1–2 days. PTH is needed for activation of renal 25-hydroxyvitamin D 1α-hydroxylase to convert 25-hydroxyvitamin D to 1,25-dihydroxyvitamin D (calcitriol). Calcitriol increases absorption of calcium from the gut and reabsorption of calcium from the skeleton. An initial dose of calcitriol is typically 0.25–0.5 mcg twice daily. Alfacalcidol is used outside the United States [1, 3, 4, 7].

The only reversible cause of hypoparathyroidism is hypomagnesemia. Magnesium is a cofactor for PTH secretion, and there can be reversible resistance to PTH when magnesium is administered and circulating PTH rapidly rises. Hypocalcemia will be difficult to correct without first normalizing the serum magnesium concentration [1, 3, 4, 7].

There are limited data on the use of PTH in patients with acute hypocalcemia. There are a few case reports using PTH(1-34) in the postoperative period after parathyroid or thyroid surgery or renal transplant [8–12]. There are no data initiating PTH therapy in patients with chronic hypoparathyroidism and acute hypocalcemia.

Outcome

This patient was given calcium carbonate 1500 mg, calcitriol 0.25 mcg, and ergocalciferol 50,000 IU in the emergency room. She was started on an intravenous calcium gluconate infusion at 50 mL per hour (10 g calcium carbonate in 1 L normal saline, approximately 50 mg/kg/h). Her repeat serum calcium level 4 hours later had increased to 8.6 mg/dL, and her calcium infusion was discontinued. She reported feeling back to her baseline with no complaints except for mild cramping of her hands which had been present since surgery. She was discharged home from the emergency room on a regimen of calcium carbonate 1000 mg three times daily, calcitriol 0.5 mcg twice day, and ergocalciferol 50,000 IU weekly for 2 months. She eventually recovered parathyroid function at approximately 7 months postoperatively, and calcium and calcitriol were discontinued at that time.

Clinical Pearls and Pitfalls

- Administration of intravenous calcium should be considered for clinical features of hypocalcemia (including broncho- or laryngospasm, tetany, seizures, prolongation of the QT interval) and/or patients with marked hypocalcemia (i.e., corrected calcium lower than 7.0 mg/dL).
- Intravenous calcium gluconate is preferred because it can be administered peripherally.
- Oral calcium should be initiated as soon possible since the effects of intravenous calcium are short.
- Hypomagnesemia should be addressed if present.

Conflict of Interest   The authors declare no conflicts of interest.

References

1. Bilezikian JP, Brandi ML, Cusano NE, Mannstadt M, Rejnmark L, Rizzoli R, Rubin MR, Winer KK, Liberman UA, Potts JT Jr. Management of hypoparathyroidism: present and future. J Clin Endocrinol Metab. 2016;101(6):2313–24.

2. Powers J, Joy K, Ruscio A, Lagast H. Prevalence and incidence of hypoparathyroidism in the United States using a large claims database. J Bone Miner Res. 2013;28(12):2570–6.
3. Brandi ML, Bilezikian JP, Shoback D, et al. Management of hypoparathyroidism: summary statement and guidelines. J Clin Endocrinol Metab. 2016;101(6):2273–83.
4. Stack BC Jr, Bimston DN, Bodenner DL, Brett EM, Dralle H, Orloff LA, Pallota J, Snyder SK, Wong RJ, Randolph GW. American association of clinical endocrinologists and American college of endocrinology disease state clinical review: postoperative hypoparathyroidism—definitions and management. Endocr Pract. 2015;21(6):674–85.
5. Fonseca OA, Calverley JR. Neurological manifestations of hypoparathyroidism. Arch Intern Med. 1967;120(2):202–6.
6. Schaaf M, Payne CA. Effect of diphenylhydantoin and phenobarbital on overt and latent tetany. N Engl J Med. 1966;274(22):1228–33.
7. Gafni RI, Collins MT. Hypoparathyroidism. N Engl J Med. 2019;380(18):1738–47.
8. Ballane GT, Sfeir JG, Dakik HA, Brown EM, El-Hajj Fuleihan G. Use of recombinant human parathyroid hormone in hypocalcemic cardiomyopathy. Eur J Endocrinol. 2012;166:1113–20.
9. Castellano K, Plantalech L. Post surgical hypoparathyroidism (HP): treatment with teriparatide (TP). Bone. 2006;38:S7.
10. Puig-Domingo M, Díaz G, Nicolau J, Fernández C, Rueda S, Halperin I. Successful treatment of vitamin D unresponsive hypoparathyroidism with multipulse subcutaneous infusion of teriparatide. Eur J Endocrinol. 2008;159:653–7.
11. Mahajan A, Narayanan M, Jaffers G, Concepcion L. Hypoparathyroidism associated with severe mineral bone disease postrenal transplantation, treated successfully with recombinant PTH. Hemodial Int. 2009;13:547–50.
12. Mishra PE, Schwartz BL, Sarafoglou K, Hook K, Kim Y, Petryk A. Short-term PTH(1-34) therapy in children to correct severe hypocalcemia and hyperphosphatemia due to hypoparathyroidism: two case studies. Case Rep Endocrinol. 2016;2016:6838626.

Chapter 2
Acute Hypocalcemia from Proton Pump Inhibitor Use

Franco Vallejo and Melissa Sum

Case Presentation

A 58-year-old woman with a history of papillary thyroid cancer status post total thyroidectomy 20 years ago with subsequent postsurgical hypothyroidism and hypoparathyroidism presented to the emergency room with severe, symptomatic hypocalcemia 4 days after starting lansoprazole.

She reported a history of well-controlled hypoparathyroidism on calcitriol 0.5 mcg once a day, daily intake of three to four servings of calcium-rich foods, and chlorthalidone for hypercalciuria. Due to recent symptoms of gastroesophageal reflux, her primary care doctor prescribed lansoprazole, a proton pump inhibitor (PPI). The patient inquired about potential interactions of this therapy with her regimen for hypoparathyroidism and was reassured against adverse effects.

F. Vallejo · M. Sum (✉)
Division of Endocrinology, Diabetes and Metabolism, Department of Internal Medicine, New York University School of Medicine, New York, NY, USA
e-mail: melissa.sum@nyulangone.org

© Springer Nature Switzerland AG 2020   9
N. E. Cusano (ed.), *Hypoparathyroidism*,
https://doi.org/10.1007/978-3-030-29433-5_2

Shortly after starting lansoprazole, she began to experience acral numbness and tingling. Four days later, she had uncontrolled locking of her extremities prompting her to go to the emergency department. Physical exam was notable for a well-healed anterior neck scar, positive Trousseau's sign, and absent Chvostek's sign.

Laboratory evaluation was notable for total serum calcium 5.9 mg/dL [8.4–10.2 mg/dL], magnesium 1.4 mg/dL [1.6–2.3 mg/dL], phosphorus 6.5 mg/dL [2.3–4.7 mg/dL], albumin 3.6 g/dL [3.5–5.2 g/dL], 25-hydroxyvitamin D 25 16 ng/mL [30–80 ng/mL], and intact PTH 5 pg/mL [15–75 pg/mL]. ECG showed mildly a prolonged corrected QT interval of 484 milliseconds.

Assessment and Diagnosis

The most likely diagnosis for a patient with hypoparathyroidism presenting with numbness, tingling, and locking is hypocalcemia, and indeed, she was diagnosed with tetany from severe symptomatic hypocalcemia. Furthermore, the hypocalcemia most likely resulted from decreased gastrointestinal calcium absorption after initiation of PPI therapy given its development a few days after lansoprazole therapy.

Postsurgical hypoparathyroidism can occur after thyroid, parathyroid, or other neck surgery and often manifests with the symptoms of hypocalcemia that include perioral numbness, hand and feet paresthesias, and muscle cramps. The prevalence of permanent postsurgical hypoparathyroidism can range from 0.8% to 3% after total thyroidectomy [1, 2]. Injury to the parathyroid glands and damage of their blood supply during thyroidectomy and incidental parathyroidectomy are independent risk factors for hypocalcemia [3]. Severe symptoms of hypocalcemia include carpopedal spasm, laryngospasm, or seizures. The mainstay of chronic management typically involves the use of calcium supplements and calcitriol or active vitamin D to maintain an adequate serum corrected calcium level.

Intestinal calcium absorption is variable, and factors that affect absorption include amount of calcium ingested, transit time in the small and large intestine, and bioavailability. Calcium absorption is pH-dependent [4, 5]. Ingested calcium reaches the stomach, where gastric acid substantially lowers the pH of stomach contents and allows for calcium to solubilize (Fig. 2.1). After the stomach contents are expelled into the small intestine, the pH increases, and a portion of the calcium reprecipitates [6, 7]. Only ionized calcium can be absorbed, and absorption occurs in the small and large colon.

PPIs are widely used and have a good safety profile. PPIs inhibit the parietal cell H + K + ATPase pump leading to suppression of acid secretion, which raises the pH in the stomach and can impair calcium absorption. Furthermore, PPIs have been associated with hypomagnesemia, with a proposed mechanism being due to gastrointestinal magnesium loss [8]. Hypocalcemia secondary to hypomagnesemia is due to functional hypoparathyroidism because parathyroid hormone release is a magnesium-dependent process [9]. This hypocalcemia is refractory to correction until the magnesium deficit has been corrected.

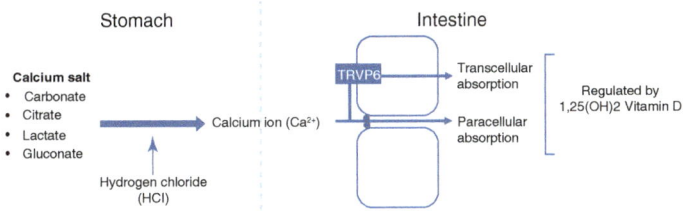

FIGURE 2.1 Intestinal calcium absorption. Calcium absorption occurs in its ionized form. Ionized calcium is formed when a dietary calcium salt reacts with HCl secreted in the stomach to dissolve. Absorption in the intestine can happen in two ways: first transcellularly through the calcium uptake channel called TRPV6 or transient receptor potential vanilloid channel type 6, which requires energy and is saturable, and second paracellularly through tight junctions, which does not require energy and is unsaturable. Both mechanisms are regulated by 1,25-dihydroxyvitamin D

In patients with hypoparathyroidism, the use of PPIs has been linked to severe hypocalcemia [10–12]. The most likely mechanism is the decrease in calcium absorption in patients with achlorhydria. In other instances, PPI usage can induce hypocalcemia by means of hypomagnesemia and its impairing effects on parathyroid hormone [13].

In our case, the patient's mildly low serum magnesium was less likely to have been a significant contribution because she already had baseline hypoparathyroidism that was effectively treated, and the main mechanism by which hypomagnesemia causes hypocalcemia is by inducing hypoparathyroidism.

Management

Her severe, symptomatic hypocalcemia required immediate treatment. She was started on intravenous calcium gluconate along with oral calcium carbonate and calcitriol. Her symptoms resolved rapidly. Her proton pump inhibitor was discontinued.

With regard to calcium supplements, calcium carbonate is a commonly used calcium salt that contains the highest percentage of elemental calcium, at 40% per weight. In comparison, calcium citrate contains 21% elemental calcium, calcium lactate 14%, and calcium gluconate 9% [14]. However, the calcium salts differ with regard to their solubility. Calcium carbonate is the least soluble salt at a neutral pH. Experiments have shown only 1% of 500 mg of calcium carbonate to dissolve in 500 ml of water after 1 hour at 37 °C. Decreasing the pH in the same experiment dissolves 86% of the calcium carbonate, and further lowering the pH to 2.5, a value observed in the stomach, increases the dissolved fraction to 100%. For this reason, calcium carbonate requires administration with food to decrease the gastric pH for improved calcium solubility, in contrast to calcium citrate, which dissolves 17 times more readily in water than calcium carbonate. Interestingly, our patient case suggests that absorption of dietary calcium can also be impacted by PPI therapy because at baseline, she ingested calcium from her diet rather than from supplements.

Since acid reflux is commonly encountered, it is important to remember that patients with hypoparathyroidism are dependent on oral calcium intake to maintain adequate serum adjusted calcium levels and caution should be administered with the use of PPIs in this population. Less potent acid-reducing medications such as histamine-2-receptor blockers (H2-blockers) can be an alternative therapy for such patients. In those patients with hypoparathyroidism who require acid-suppressive therapy, appropriate discussion of the risks and signs of hypocalcemia is advised as well as consideration of adding a more soluble calcium salt such as calcium citrate to the regimen.

Outcome

As an outpatient, she remained off lansoprazole and on a stable regimen of calcitriol, calcium carbonate, and chlorthalidone.

Clinical Pearls and Pitfalls
- Proton pump inhibitor (PPI) therapy can induce severe, symptomatic hypocalcemia in patients with chronic hypoparathyroidism.
- PPIs have been associated with hypomagnesemia, and this can induce hypocalcemia. Both hypomagnesemia and hypocalcemia should be treated simultaneously.
- H2-blockers can be an alternative therapy in patients with gastroesophageal reflux disease (GERD) and chronic hypoparathyroidism.
- Consideration should be taken regarding the addition of a more soluble calcium salt such as calcium citrate to the regimen in patients with hypoparathyroidism who require PPI therapy.
- If PPI therapy is required in a patient with hypoparathyroidism, it should be limited to the shortest duration and lowest effective dose with appropriate patient education.

Conflict of Interest   The authors declare no conflicts of interest.

References

1. Hundahl SA, Cady B, Cunningham MP, Mazzaferri E, McKee RF, Rosai J, Shah JP, Fremgen AM, Stewart AK, Holzer S. Initial results from a prospective cohort study of 5583 cases of thyroid carcinoma treated in the United States during 1996. U.S. and German Thyroid Cancer Study Group. An American College of Surgeons Commission on Cancer Patient Care Evaluation study. Cancer. 2000;89(1):202.
2. Rafferty MA, Goldstein DP, Rotstein L, Asa SL, Panzarella T, Gullane P, Gilbert RW, Brown DH, Irish JC. Completion thyroidectomy versus total thyroidectomy: is there a difference in complication rates? An analysis of 350 patients. J Am Coll Surg. 2007;205(4):602.
3. Abboud B, et al. Risk factors for postthyroidectomy hypocalcemia. J Am Coll Surg. 2002;195:456–61.
4. Recker RR. Calcium absorption and achlorhydria. N Engl J Med. 1985;313(2):70–3.
5. Graziani G, Como G, Badalamenti S, et al. Effect of gastric acid secretion on intestinal phosphate and calcium absorption in normal subjects. Nephrol Dial Transplant. 1995;10(8):1376–80.
6. Bronner F, Pansu D. Nutritional aspects of calcium absorption. J Nutr. 1999;129(1):9–12.
7. Axelson J, Persson P, Gagnemo-Persson R, Håkanson R. Importance of the stomach in maintaining calcium homoeostasis in the rat. Gut. 1991;32(11):1298–302.
8. Ito T, Jensen RT. Association of long-term proton pump inhibitor therapy with bone fractures and effects on absorption of calcium, vitamin B12, iron, and magnesium. Curr Gastroenterol Rep. 2010;12:448.
9. Sivakumar J. Proton pump inhibitor-induced hypomagnesaemia and hypocalcaemia: case review. Int J Physiol Pathophysiol Pharmacol. 2016;8(4):169–74.
10. Milman S, Epstein EJ. Proton pump inhibitor-induced hypocalcemic seizure in a patient with hypoparathyroidism. Endocr Pract. 2011;17(1):104–7.
11. Subbiah V, Tayek JA. Tetany secondary to the use of a proton-pump inhibitor. Ann Intern Med. 2002;137(3):219.

12. Zaya NE, Woodson G. Proton pump inhibitor suppression of calcium absorption presenting as respiratory distress in a patient with bilateral laryngeal paralysis and hypocalcemia. Ear Nose Throat J. 2010;89(2):78–80.
13. Epstein M, McGrath S, Law F. Proton-pump inhibitors and hypomagnesemic hypoparathyroidism. N Engl J Med. 2006;355(17):1834–6.
14. Kopic S, Geibel JP. Gastric acid, calcium absorption, and their impact on bone health. Physiol Rev. 2013;93:189–268.

Chapter 3
Conventional Therapy of Hypoparathyroidism

E. Pauline Liao

Case Presentation

A 48-year-old man with a history of kidney stones was diagnosed with primary hyperparathyroidism. Bone density was within the normal range, and he had no history of fractures. He underwent uneventful removal of 3 ½ parathyroid glands for parathyroid hyperplasia and was discharged home the following morning. Upon discharge, his calcium level was normal at 9.1 mg/dL (8.6–10.5 mg/dL), but at home he developed paresthesias. He went to urgent care, where calcium was 8.2 mg/dL with a relatively low parathyroid hormone of 15 pg/mL (14–65 pg/mL). Other testing demonstrated a 25-hydroxyvitamin D of 27.6 ng/dL (30–100 ng/mL), albumin of 4.6 g/dL (3.3–5.0), magnesium 2.0 mg/dL (1.6–2.6 mg/dL), phosphorus 5.3 mg/dL (2.5–4.5), and stage 2 chronic kidney disease (BUN/creatinine 19/1.28 mg/dL, eGFR 65 mL/min). He was initially started on calcium carbonate 1250 mg four

E. P. Liao (✉)
Department of Medicine, Division of Endocrinology,
Northwell Health/Lenox Hill Hospital, New York, NY, USA
e-mail: eliao@northwell.edu

© Springer Nature Switzerland AG 2020
N. E. Cusano (ed.), *Hypoparathyroidism*,
https://doi.org/10.1007/978-3-030-29433-5_3

17

times daily, vitamin D 400 IU daily, and calcitriol 0.25 μg three times daily. Physical examination was remarkable only for a positive Chvostek's sign and a well-healing neck incision. His serum calcium improved on this regimen to 8.7 mg/dL with a persistently low PTH concentration of 12 pg/mL. His regimen was titrated over the next few months to calcium carbonate 500 mg twice daily and calcitriol 0.25 μg twice daily. At 6 months postoperatively, laboratory testing was significant for albumin-adjusted calcium 9.1 mg/dL, PTH 10 pg/mL, 25-hydroxyvitamin D 33.8 ng/mL, phosphorus 5.3 mg/dL, magnesium 2.0 mg/dL, and BUN/creatinine 22/1.42 mg/dL (eGFR 58 mL/min). He was feeling well and only had occasional paresthesias after intense exercise; review of systems was otherwise negative.

Assessment and Diagnosis

Hypoparathyroidism is diagnosed when parathyroid hormone is undetectable or inappropriately low in the setting of hypocalcemia. Calcium should be corrected for albumin if low. Hypocalcemia (or normal serum calcium in the setting of requirement for supplementation with calcium and/or active vitamin D) with low PTH should be confirmed on at least two occasions at least 14 days apart. The most common cause of hypoparathyroidism is due to postsurgical complications of thyroid, parathyroid, or radical neck surgery for head/neck cancer. Hypoparathyroidism is transient in approximately 75% of cases, defined as lasting less than 6 months. Serum magnesium should be addressed if abnormal, since the only reversible causes of hypoparathyroidism are disorders of magnesium due to impaired secretion and resistance to PTH [1]. Chronic hypoparathyroidism, defined as lasting 6 months or greater, complicates approximately 1–5% of all anterior neck surgeries [2, 3]. Other causes of hypoparathyroidism include autoimmune and genetic disorders and will be discussed in the subsequent chapters. The First International Workshop on the Management of Hypoparathyroidism [4] provides the following guidelines for initial evaluation of a patient with hypoparathyroidism:

1. Historical aspects: family history; personal history of anterior neck surgery; gastrointestinal, renal, and skeletal review for gastrointestinal symptoms, renal stones, and fractures, respectively; general quality of life; and medications and supplements.
2. Physical examination, key elements: eye examination for cataracts and calcifications, anterior neck for signs of previous surgery, signs of neuromuscular irritability (Chvostek's, Trousseau's sign), nail beds for fungal infection, mucosal candidiasis, range of motion of joints, and the skin for vitiligo.

Management

There are statements from the European Society of Endocrinology [5] and the First International Workshop on the Management of Hypoparathyroidism [4] to provide guidance in management of patients with hypoparathyroidism. The goals of chronic hypoparathyroidism management are to prevent signs and symptoms of hypocalcemia; maintain serum calcium in the low-normal range, or within 0.5 mg/dL of the lower limit of the normal range; maintain the calcium-phosphate product below 55 mg^2/dL^2 (4.4 $mmol^2/L^2$); avoid hypercalciuria; and avoid development of nephrolithiasis and other extraskeletal calcifications. Treatment should be personalized to focus on overall well-being and quality of life [4].

Calcium carbonate is the most commonly used form of calcium supplementation because it contains 40% elemental calcium and is the least expensive formulation. However, since it requires an acidic environment for optimal absorption, for individuals with achlorhydria or who are taking proton pump inhibitors, calcium citrate is more effective, though it contains only 21% elemental calcium. The typical oral calcium supplementation is 0.5–1 g of elemental calcium 2–4 per day, but requirements vary widely, with some patients requiring very high doses of calcium [4]. Calcium must be taken throughout the day to maintain serum calcium. Certain "natural" forms of calcium can contain lead [6]. Patients may require additional calcium during acute infection, with exercise, or at times of stress [7].

Active vitamin D (1,25-dihydroxyvitamin D, calcitriol) promotes bone remodeling and increases intestinal calcium absorption. Patients with hypoparathyroidism have impaired activation of vitamin D since PTH stimulates the renal 1-alpha-hydroxylase. Calcitriol is the most common vitamin D supplementation used because it is the most active metabolite of vitamin D, does not require renal activation, and is also the least expensive formulation available. It has a rapid onset of action (hours) and short half-life (4–6 hours), in case hypercalcemia develops [8]. The typical calcitriol dose is between 0.25 and 2 µg per day. If the total dose is greater than 0.75–1.0 µg per day, it is recommended to use divided doses [9]. Other synthetic vitamin D analogs are available (alfacalcidol, dihydrotachysterol) outside the United States. The typical dose for alfacalcidol is 0.5–3.0 µg daily. A higher active vitamin D dose can be used to reduce calcium supplementation.

Magnesium and vitamin D deficiencies should also be corrected [4, 5]. In patients with some residual parathyroid function, magnesium is an important cofactor in parathyroid hormone secretion. The symptoms of hypomagnesemia are also similar to those of hypocalcemia. The guidelines recommend therapy with parent vitamin D (ergo- or cholecalciferol) to maintain 25-hydroxyvitamin D at least 20 ng/mL or above, even if the patient is treated with active vitamin D. The half-life of parent vitamin D is 2–3 weeks, and some experts feel that it may help provide smoother control of serum calcium in the setting of the short half-life of calcitriol. Extrarenal production of 1-alpha-hydroxylase is another possible source of 1,25-dihydroxyvitamin D. Vitamin D has effects on muscle function and may also have other extraskeletal effects, which is an area of active investigation.

For patients with hyperphosphatemia, decreasing the ratio of calcitriol to calcium may be helpful. Calcitriol increases intestinal absorption of both calcium and phosphorus, while calcium can act as a phosphate binder. A low-phosphate diet may be helpful in some patients [4]. No data exist on the use of phosphate binders in patients with hypoparathyroidism.

Serum calcium, phosphate, magnesium, and eGFR should be monitored regularly and more frequently during dosing adjustments (every 1–4 weeks). The European guidelines recommend biochemical monitoring every 3–6 months [5], with the international guidelines recommending at least annually [4]. The 24-hour urine calcium should also be measured periodically to ensure the patient is not developing hypercalciuria, every 1–2 years per the guidelines. A thiazide diuretic can be added in patients who develop hypercalciuria (24-hour urine calcium >250 mg for women or >300 mg/24 h for men), in conjunction with a low sodium diet. High diuretic doses are often required for control of hypercalciuria. Renal imaging, ophthalmologic examination for cataracts, central nervous system imaging for basal ganglia or other calcifications, and bone density testing can be considered as clinically indicated [4, 5].

Parathyroid hormone [rhPTH(1–84), Natpara] became available in 2015 for patients who are difficult to control on conventional therapy. Not all patients with hypoparathyroidism are candidates for rhPTH(1–84), which will be discussed in the following chapter.

Outcome

His regimen for hypoparathyroidism was adjusted to calcium citrate 500 mg three times daily (changed from calcium carbonate due to taking a proton pump inhibitor for gastric reflux) and calcitriol 0.25 μg daily. He was encouraged to have additional calcium supplementation prior to intense exercise. The patient has no symptoms of hypoparathyroidism on his current regimen. Serum calcium has been maintained in the

8.4–8.9 mg/dL range, and phosphate declined to 4.5 mg/dL. The 24-hour urine calcium excretion was ordered and was 170 mg/24 h, within the sex-specific range. Renal ultrasound was negative for calcification. He is followed every 6 months with biochemical testing prior to office visits.

Clinical Pitfalls and Pearls

- Patients are prone to both hypercalcemia and hypocalcemia.
- Calcium supplementation needs to be administered in divided doses and throughout the day to maintain serum calcium levels.
- Calcium carbonate contains 40% elemental calcium and is optimally dosed around mealtimes, since it requires acid for absorption. For patients on proton pump inhibitors or with achlorhydria, calcium citrate (21% elemental calcium) is a more reliable option.
- Calcitriol can be increased to reduce calcium supplementation but should be reduced in patients with hyperphosphatemia.
- Regular monitoring should include serum magnesium, phosphate, eGFR, and 24-hour urine calcium, in addition to serum calcium.

Conflict of Interest   The authors declare no conflicts of interest.

References

1. Clarke BL, Brown EM, Collins MT, Jüppner H, Lakatos P, Levine MA, Mannstadt MM, Bilezikian JP, Romanischen AF, Thakker RV. Epidemiology and diagnosis of hypoparathyroidism. J Clin Endocrinol Metab. 2016;101(6):2284–99.

2. Powers J, Joy K, Ruscio A, Lagast H. Prevalence and incidence of hypoparathyroidism in the United States using a large claims database. J Bone Miner Res. 2013;28(12):2570–6.
3. Mannstadt M, Bilezikian JP, Thakker RV, Hannan FM, Clarke BL, Rejnmark L, et al. Hypoparathyroidism. Nat Rev Dis Primers. 2017;3:17080.
4. Brandi ML, Bilezikian JP, Shoback D, et al. Management of hypoparathyroidism: summary statement and guidelines. J Clin Endocrinol Metab. 2016;101(6):2273–83.
5. Bollerslev J, Rejnmark L, Marcocci C, Shoback DM, Sitges-Serra A, van Biesen W, et al. European Society of Endocrinology Clinical Guideline: treatment of chronic hypoparathyroidism in adults. Eur J Endocrinol. 2015;173(2):G1–G20.
6. Scelfo GM, Flegal AR. Lead in calcium supplements. Environ Health Perspect. 2000;108(4):309–19.
7. Sinnott B. Hypoparathyroidism—review of the literature. J Rare Dis Diagn Ther. 2018;4(3):12.
8. Gafni RI, Collins MT. Hypoparathyroidism. N Engl J Med. 2019;380(18):1738–47.
9. Stack BC Jr, Bimston DN, Bodenner DL, Brett EM, Dralle H, Orloff LA, Pallota J, Snyder SK, Wong RJ, Randolph GW. American association of clinical endocrinologists and american college of endocrinology disease state clinical review: postoperative hypoparathyroidism – definitions and management. Endocr Pract. 2015;21(6):674–85.

Chapter 4
Treatment with Parathyroid Hormone

Natalie E. Cusano and John P. Bilezikian

Case Presentation

A 23-year-old woman with a history of compressive goiter status post-total thyroidectomy 1 year ago with postsurgical hypoparathyroidism is now transferring her care. The pathology report from her surgery showed Hashimoto's disease with no evidence of cancer and one parathyroid gland. Her postoperative course was complicated by hypocalcemia, requiring hospitalization of almost 1 week. She has had persistent hypoparathyroidism and trouble maintaining her calcium level at goal, with six emergency department visits since diagnosis. She describes waking up every day with perioral

N. E. Cusano (✉)
Department of Medicine, Division of Endocrinology,
Northwell Health/Lenox Hill Hospital, New York, NY, USA
e-mail: ncusano@northwell.edu

J. P. Bilezikian
Department of Medicine, Division of Endocrinology,
College of Physicians & Surgeons, Columbia University, New York, NY, USA

© Springer Nature Switzerland AG 2020
N. E. Cusano (ed.), *Hypoparathyroidism*,
https://doi.org/10.1007/978-3-030-29433-5_4

and extremity numbness and tingling, with intermittent symptoms present during the day.

Her regimen for hypoparathyroidism includes calcium citrate 1200 mg three times daily, calcitriol 1.0 µg twice daily, a serving of yogurt with breakfast, and vitamin D 10,000 IU weekly. Her other medications include levothyroxine 112 mcg daily and a combined oral contraceptive pill. She reports compliance with all medications. Physical examination is unremarkable, other than negative Chvostek's sign and well-healed neck incision with no palpable thyroid tissue. Laboratory evaluation was significant for calcium 8.4 mg/dL (normal: 8.7–10.2; 2.10 mmol/L; corrected for serum albumin), PTH 5 pg/mL (15–65; 5 ng/L), 25-hydroxyvitamin D 34.0 ng/mL (>30 ng/mL; 85 nmol/L), BUN/creatinine 13/0.5 mg/dL (eGFR 154 mL/min), phosphorus 4.8 mg/dL (2.5–4.5; 1.55 mmol/L), magnesium 1.6 mg/dL (1.6–2.6; 0.80 mmol/L), and 24-hour urine calcium 407 mg (100–250; 10.2 mmol). Renal ultrasound was negative for nephrocalcinosis or stone.

Assessment and Diagnosis

While only one parathyroid gland was removed at the time of total thyroidectomy, the symptomatic hypocalcemia with virtually undetectable PTH level leads to several possible conclusions. One possibility is that all four glands were actually removed although the pathological examination only reported one in the specimen. Without an exhaustive investigation of parathyroid tissue in pathological specimens, the glands in the specimen could have been missed. Another possibility is that the postoperative hypoparathyroidism is due to permanent damage to the remaining parathyroid glands by virtue of their vascular supply being compromised. Sometimes this is a transient state, but since it has been a year since her neck surgery, one must assume that she has chronic hypoparathyroidism. Chronic hypoparathyroidism is defined by time, namely, post neck surgery of at least 6 months.

A change in her regimen is warranted since she is often symptomatic of hypocalcemia. One would be reluctant to increase her regimen of calcium and calcitriol even further because her current regimen already exceeds the guidelines for management (see below). Recombinant human PTH(1–84), rhPTH(1–84) (Natpara, Natpar), was approved by the Food and Drug Administration in 2015 for the treatment of "patients who cannot be well-controlled on calcium supplements and active forms of vitamin D alone" [1]. rhPTH(1–84) received similar approval from the European Medicines Agency in 2017. Until approval of rhPTH(1–84), hypoparathyroidism was the only classic endocrine deficiency disease for which the replacement hormone was not an approved treatment. Approval of once-daily subcutaneous rhPTH(1–84) was based on data from the pivotal REPLACE trial demonstrating a decrease in calcium and calcitriol requirements in the treatment arm while serum calcium was maintained [2]. The specific end points of the study were a >50% reduction in baseline calcium and calcitriol requirements while maintaining the serum calcium within the normal range. Relative to the control group who received placebo injections, those receiving rhPTH(1–84) responded in a highly significant manner.

The First International Workshop on the Management of Hypoparathyroidism provides guidance regarding patients who may fall under the category of being difficult to control [3]. The guidelines recommend consideration of rhPTH(1–84) therapy for the following indications: (1) inadequate control of the serum calcium concentration; (2) calcium requirements >2.5 g and/or active vitamin D >1.5 mcg daily; (3) hypercalciuria, renal stones, nephrocalcinosis, stone risk, or reduced creatinine clearance or eGFR (<60 mL/min); (4) hyperphosphatemia and/or calcium-phosphate product >55 mg^2/dL^2 (4.4 $mmol^2/L^2$); (5) a gastrointestinal tract disorder associated with malabsorption; and/or (6) reduced quality of life. This patient clearly meets the indications of inadequate control of serum calcium, high calcium and calcitriol requirements, hypercalciuria, and hyperphosphatemia.

While other treatment decisions can be considered, this patient would be expected to benefit most from rhPTH(1–84) therapy. Increasing calcium or calcitriol further would likely worsen her hypercalciuria, and she is already taking high doses of both. Hydrochlorothiazide may be helpful for hypercalciuria; however, therapy with hydrochlorothiazide would not be expected to ameliorate her symptoms.

Management

The starting dose of rhPTH(1–84) is 50 μg daily and can be titrated to 25, 75, or 100 μg daily as needed [1]. Of note, rhPTH(1–84) was recalled in September 2019 due to issues with the delivery device but not the medication itself. rhPTH(1–84) should be administered subcutaneously into the thigh due to pharmacokinetic data showing increased duration of effect over delivery from the abdomen. Patients should be instructed to decrease calcitriol by 50% when starting rhPTH(1–84). Serum calcium should be monitored 3–7 days after treatment initiation, with further titration of supplemental calcitriol or calcium as needed [3]. rhPTH(1–84) has not been formally studied in cases of acute postoperative hypocalcemia or in patients with calcium-sensing receptor mutations. Also of note is that rhPTH(1–84) is pregnancy Category C risk, with animal reproductive studies showing adverse effects but no adequate and well-controlled studies in humans [1].

Providers prescribing rhPTH(1–84) and patients starting therapy must be enrolled in the Risk Evaluation and Mitigation Strategy (REMS) program to monitor risk for osteosarcoma. Osteosarcoma, a bone cancer, has been noted in rats given very high doses of PTH and PTH analogs for a very long period of time (2 rat years is generally equivalent to 75 human years of life). Caution should be used in patients at increased risk of osteosarcoma, including those with a history of radiation therapy and children with open epiphyses. There have been no adverse signals of osteosarcoma in humans treated with any form of PTH [4, 5]. Data are now available in hypoparathyroid patients treated with rhPTH(1–84) through eight years [6]. Since rhPTH(1–84) will likely be used indefinitely, further long-term data are needed. Management must be personalized to balance symptoms with the risks of treatment. Most experts do not feel that osteosarcoma presents a clear risk in human subjects. With teriparatide, the foreshortened analog of PTH(1–84), surveillance for over 16 years has not resulted in any human safety signals in this regard. Given that rhPTH(1–84) will be used for more than the 2 years that teriparatide and abaloparatide are used for the treatment of osteoporosis, the safety surveillance program is appropriate.

Once-daily subcutaneous rhPTH(1–84) was not demonstrated to decrease urine calcium excretion in the 6-month REPLACE trial, although data from the open-label extension of the prior RACE trial did show reduction in urinary calcium over time [7]. Other studies have shown a gradual reduction in urinary calcium excretion with the long-term use of rhPTH(1–84) [6]. Further studies are needed to determine if rhPTH(1–84) can decrease the risk of renal complications or development of extraskeletal calcifications. Different treatment paradigms and products have also been studied. PTH(1–34) has been studied in children and adults with hypoparathyroidism, although twice or thrice daily dosing is usually necessary to provide control of serum calcium [8, 9]. It is not clear why more frequent dosing of teriparatide is required in view of the similar half-lives of both teriparatide and rhPTH(1–84) in the circulation. The longer effective half-life of rhPTH(1–84) might be related to pharmacokinetics of uptake at the site of injection or to longer biological effects of rhPTH(1–84). Winer and colleagues published preliminary data using a more physiologic replacement regimen of continuous PTH(1–34) administration by pump demonstrating a 59% reduction in urine calcium excretion in patients with postsurgical hypoparathyroidism [10]. It is important to note that the use of PTH(1–34) in hypoparathyroidism in the United States remains off-label. The PARALLAX study of twice daily rhPTH(1–84) dosing (NCT02781844) was completed, but results are not yet published. TransCon PTH is an inactive prodrug of PTH(1–34) bound to a carrier that provides free PTH at a steady state with an infusion-like profile [11]. Phase 1 study results were presented demonstrating safety in healthy patients and a drug half-life of 60 hours, with plans for a phase 2 study.

Outcome

The patient was started on rhPTH(1–84) 50 μg daily with decrease in her calcitriol dose by 50%. She was carefully monitored and eventually titrated to rhPTH(1–84) 100 μg daily. With this higher dose, she no longer requires supplementation with calcium and calcitriol. She continues to take a serving of yogurt in the morning. She no longer has hypocalcemic symptoms. Her 24-hour urine calcium remained elevated, and she was started on hydrochlorothiazide 50 mg and amiloride 5 mg daily in addition to a low sodium diet, with improvement in urine calcium excretion to within the sex-specific normal range.

Clinical Pearls and Pitfalls

- rhPTH(1–84) is indicated for patients with hypoparathyroidism that is difficult to control with conventional therapy.
- rhPTH(1–84) is started at a dose of 50 μg subcutaneously daily with titration to 25, 75, or 100 μg daily as needed.
- Calcitriol should be decreased by 50% when starting rhPTH(1–84), with close monitoring of serum calcium and additional adjustment in supplementation as needed.
- More data are needed regarding whether treatment with PTH therapy can decrease the risk of complications of hypoparathyroidism.

Conflict of Interest   The authors declare no conflicts of interest.

References

1. Natpara [package insert]. Available at: https://www.accessdata. fda.gov/drugsatfda_docs/label/2015/125511s000lbl.pdf.
2. Mannstadt M, Clarke BL, Vokes T, et al. Efficacy and safety of recombinant human parathyroid hormone (1-84) in hypoparathyroidism (REPLACE): a double-blind, placebo-controlled, randomised, phase 3 study. Lancet Diabetes Endocrinol. 2013;1:275–83.
3. Brandi ML, Bilezikian JP, Shoback D, Bouillon R, Clarke BL, Thakker RV, Khan AA, Potts JT Jr. Management of hypoparathyroidism: summary statement and guidelines. J Clin Endocrinol Metab. 2016;101(6):2273–83.
4. Andrews EB, Gilsenan AW, Midkiff K, Sherrill B, Wu Y, Mann BH, Masica D. The US postmarketing surveillance study of adult osteosarcoma and teriparatide: study design and findings from the first 7 years. J Bone Miner Res. 2012;27(12):2429–37.
5. Cipriani C, Irani D, Bilezikian JP. Safety of osteoanabolic therapy: a decade of experience. J Bone Miner Res. 2012;27(12):2419–28.
6. Tay YD, Tabacco G, Cusano NE, Williams J, Omeragic B, Majeed R, Almonte MG, Bilezikian JP, Rubin MR. Therapy of Hypoparathyroidism with rhPTH(1–84): A Prospective Eight Year Investigation of Efficacy and Safety. J Clin Endocrinol Metab. 2019 [Epub ahead of print].
7. Bilezikian JP, Bone HG, Clarke BL, et al. Safety and efficacy of recombinant human parathyroid hormone 1–84 for the treatment of adults with chronic hypoparathyroidism: six-year results of the RACE study. Presented at ENDO 2019, New Orleans. Available at: https://www.abstractsonline.com/pp8/#!/5752/presentation/16334.
8. Winer KK, Ko CW, Reynolds JC, et al. Long-term treatment of hypoparathyroidism: a randomized controlled study comparing parathyroid hormone-(1-34) versus calcitriol and calcium. J Clin Endocrinol Metab. 2003;88:4214–20.
9. Winer KK, Kelly A, Johns A, Zhang B, et al. Long-term parathyroid hormone 1-34 replacement therapy in children with hypoparathyroidism. J Pediatr. 2018;203:391–9.
10. Winer KK, Zhang B, Shrader JA, et al. Synthetic human parathyroid hormone 1-34 replacement therapy: a randomized crossover trial comparing pump versus injections in the treatment of chronic hypoparathyroidism. J Clin Endocrinol Metab. 2012;97:391–9.
11. Karpf D, Mortensen E, Sprogøe K, et al. The design and preliminary results of a phase 1 TransCon PTH trial in healthy volunteers. Endocr Abstr. 2018;56:GP174.

Chapter 5
Autoimmune Hypoparathyroidism

Kelly L. Roszko and Rachel I. Gafni

Case Presentation

The patient was the 9-pound, 21-inch product of an uncomplicated pregnancy. His mother noted that he was a poor nurser, lethargic and listless at times, weighing only 11 pounds at 6 months of age. After switching to formula, he began to thrive and grew well until 7 years of age, at which point his growth slowed again and he was reported to have steatorrhea. At 2.5 years, he began to suffer from dry skin, patchy alopecia, and frequent mucocutaneous fungal infections. At age 9, laboratory studies were obtained because of a 1-year history of sporadic symptoms including fatigue, leg and hand cramps, double vision, and occasional difficulty breathing. Blood calcium was 5.3 mg/dL (8.5–10.5), with a phosphorus of 10.9 mg/dL (3.5–6) and an undetectable PTH. Concurrent with the diagnosis of hypocalcemia, he developed primary

K. L. Roszko · R. I. Gafni (✉)
Skeletal Disorders and Mineral Homeostasis Section,
National Institutes of Dental and Craniofacial Research,
National Institutes of Health, Bethesda, MD, USA
e-mail: gafnir@nidcr.nih.gov

© Springer Nature Switzerland AG 2020
N. E. Cusano (ed.), *Hypoparathyroidism*,
https://doi.org/10.1007/978-3-030-29433-5_5

varicella-zoster virus (VZV) infection and presented with tetany. He was the third of five children, all of whom contracted primary VZV. The two eldest also developed tetany, with calcium measurements of 4.3 mg/dL and 5.1 mg/dL; on exam, they both had oral thrush. One of these siblings had a history of seizure disorder and basal ganglia calcifications that had been detected on a prior CT scan but had no known history of hypocalcemia.

The patient was admitted to the hospital for management of his hypocalcemia and VZV infection. He underwent a cosyntropin stimulation test which peaked at a cortisol level of 6.7 mcg/dL (normal >20) at 60 minutes, suggesting adrenal insufficiency. However, he was being treated for chronic fungal infections with ketoconazole, which can suppress adrenal steroid production. After withholding ketoconazole for 1 week, a repeat cosyntropin stimulation test peaked at a cortisol level of 20.8 mcg/dL, an adequate response. Thyroid function tests were normal. In addition, he had several large, bulky, foamy, foul-smelling stools, but neither the patient nor the mother could provide an adequate dietary history, and the cause of his steatorrhea was unclear at the time.

Assessment and Diagnosis

Insufficient PTH in the setting of hypocalcemia is diagnostic of hypoparathyroidism. Symptoms of hypocalcemia can range from mild (e.g., perioral numbness and muscle cramps), to tetany or papilledema, to severe (e.g., seizures, refractory heart failure, or laryngospasm) [1]. Hypoparathyroidism can be acquired or be part of a genetic disorder. Hypoparathyroidism in adults is most commonly due to postsurgical complications of neck surgery. Other acquired causes of hypoparathyroidism include altered serum magnesium, infiltrative diseases, and autoimmunity to the parathyroid glands. Autoimmune acquired non-monogenic hypoparathyroidism is presumed to be caused either by autoimmune destruction of the parathyroid glands or by antibodies targeting the calcium-sensing receptor (CaSR). In most patients, the action of these CaSR autoantibodies is unclear [2–4], although a positive response to immunomodulatory therapy in a patient with activating CaSR autoantibodies was recently reported [5]. In addition, the presence of these antibodies, when testing is available, is not diagnostic, and, therefore, acquired autoimmune hypoparathyroidism is a diagnosis of exclusion. This form of acquired autoimmune hypoparathyroidism may be associated with other autoimmune diseases [6]. While there is no clear genetic etiology, there is evidence to suggest that this condition may be HLA-associated [7].

Autoimmune hypoparathyroidism can also be monogenic, due to pathogenic inactivating variants in the *AIRE* gene, resulting in autoimmune polyendocrinopathy-candidiasis-ectodermal dystrophy (APECED) [also known as autoimmune polyglandular syndrome type 1 (APS1) or polyglandular autoimmune (PGA) syndrome type 1]. The vast majority of disease-causing *AIRE* variants are biallelic. The AIRE protein is expressed in the thymus, where it decreases autoimmunity. AIRE stimulates expression of peripheral tissue antigens in the thymic medullary epithelial cells, thus promoting tolerance by immune cells. In thymic medullary epithelial cells lacking AIRE, there was reduced expression of these peripheral antigens [8]. AIRE has been shown to augment regulatory T cells and decrease effector T cells. In AIRE-deficient mice, there is an increase in peripheral IL-17 producing effector T cells [9].

In this vignette, the child suffered from frequent mucocutaneous fungal infections, which, along with hypoparathyroidism and adrenal insufficiency, make up the classic triad of APECED. A clinical diagnosis is made when two elements of the classic triad are present or one disorder with a sibling who has APECED. Other manifestations include hypothyroidism, ovarian/testicular failure, growth hormone deficiency, and type 1 diabetes, as well as nonendocrine diseases including urticarial eruption, enamel hypoplasia, intestinal malabsorption, autoimmune hepatitis, autoimmune pneumonitis, autoimmune gastritis, Sjogren's-like syndrome, B12 deficiency, vitiligo, keratoconjunctivitis, alopecia, tubulointerstitial nephritis, and asplenia, which are also associated with APECED (Table 5.1)

[10, 11]. It was recently shown that APECED was diagnosed a mean of 4 years earlier when urticarial eruption, enamel hypoplasia, and intestinal malabsorption were added to the diagnostic criteria. The use of these extended diagnostic criteria was also found to avoid adrenal crisis or hypocalcemic seizure in half of the patients [11]. Early diagnosis is important, as 7 of the 52 patients in a Norwegian cohort died during childhood prior to diagnosis [12]. Hypoparathyroidism is the first and most prevalent endocrinopathy of the syndrome, typically presenting before age 10 years, with adrenal insufficiency a close second. The other endocrinopathies tend to occur at much lower rates (Table 5.1) [10]. There are slight variations in the presentations of APECED among different geographical populations, and the American patients appear to be enriched for nonendocrine manifestations [11]. APECED patients can have an increased mortality from adrenal crisis, hypocalcemic crisis, and malignancy [12].

Genetic testing for pathogenic *AIRE* variants is commercially available; however, large deletions or intronic variants might be missed, so normal sequencing does not rule out disease. The presence of interferon-α2 and interferon-ω autoantibodies is highly sensitive and specific for APECED [13, 14]; however, these tests are not widely available outside of research laboratories. Similarly, antibodies to CaSR and NALP5 have been frequently found in APECED patients [15, 16]. While parathyroid suppression by activating CaSR autoantibodies has been reported in a very small proportion of patients [17], in most patients with APECED, it appears that the CaSR autoantibodies are not activating [16]. Other autoantibodies that may be present in APECED include those against the thyroid, 21-hydroxylase, intrinsic factor, tryptophan hydroxylase, and several cytokines [11, 18]. Of note, there are many other genetic causes of hypoparathyroidism, both isolated and syndromic, that should be considered in children and adults presenting with nonsurgical hypoparathyroidism. Examples include pathogenic variants in *CASR*, *GNA11*, *GCM2*, *GATA3*, *TBCE*, and the *PTH* gene itself, as well as a chromosomal deletion of chromosome 22q11.2, an X-linked rearrangement with chromosome 2, and mitochondrial disorders [6].

TABLE 5.1 Disease manifestations of APECED in an American cohort ($n = 35$)

	Manifestation	% of American cohort with disease	Age by which disease presented
Endocrine	Hypoparathyroidism	91%	30
	Adrenal insufficiency	83%	40
	Hypothyroidism	23%	60+
	Ovarian failure	38%	20
	Testicular failure	21%	60+
	Growth hormone deficiency	17%	15
	Type 1 diabetes	11%	20
Nonendocrine oral disease	Chronic mucocutaneous candidiasis	86%	30
	Enamel hypoplasia	86%	30
Skin/nail	Urticarial eruption	66%	20
	Nail dystrophy	17%	20
	Alopecia	17%	15
	Vitiligo	37%	60+
Gastrointestinal	Intestinal dysfunction	80%	20
	Autoimmune gastritis	49%	60+
	B12 deficiency	29%	40
	Autoimmune hepatitis	43%	40

(continued)

TABLE 5.1 (continued)

	Manifestation	% of American cohort with disease	Age by which disease presented
Other	Interstitial nephritis	6%	30
	Asplenia	9%	30
	Pneumonitis	40%	50
	Keratoconjunctivitis	29%	40
	Sjogren's-like disease	43%	60+
	Early hypertension	17%	40

Adapted from Ferre et al. [11]

Management

Management of patients with APECED should be based on the presenting symptoms of the patient. In addition, involvement of a multidisciplinary team and appropriate screening for the development of other components of the disease is important. Hypoparathyroidism should be treated with calcium and calcitriol with the goal of achieving a blood calcium level in the low-normal range. Care should be taken to avoid overtreatment with calcium, which might elevate the urinary calcium and place the patient at risk for renal stones and nephrocalcinosis. In patients with significant enteropathy, absorption of calcium and calcitriol may be poor or erratic. In some, immunosuppressive agents may reduce malabsorption [10, 19]. Anecdotally, we have found that treatment with high doses of calciferol is sometimes more effective than calcitriol in preventing hypocalcemia in patients with enteropathy, as calciferols have a longer half-life than activated vitamin D; in these cases, intermittent bouts of severe malabsorption may be less associated with acute drops in vitamin D levels when using long-acting calciferols. Subcutaneous PTH may also be considered in those with refractory hypocalcemia [20, 21], although long-term safety has not been established. Addison's disease should be treated with hydrocortisone and fludrocortisone, and patients should be counseled about manifestations of adrenal insufficiency, wear a medical alert bracelet, and have a supply of stress dose steroids. Treatment of chronic mucocutaneous candidiasis typically begins with azole medications such as ketoconazole or amphotericin B oral suspension, but it can be complicated by resistant organisms. Care should be taken when using ketoconazole as it also decreases the synthesis of cortisol in the adrenal glands, which could exacerbate any looming adrenal insufficiency [22]. While immunosuppressive medications are not routinely used to treat APECED, they can be used in patients with disease in the lungs, liver, kidneys, small intestine, or eyes [10].

Continued surveillance of these patients is crucial, as additional manifestations develop over time. Interestingly, many of the associated diseases either present by age 15–30 or do not develop later in life [11] (Table 5.1). In a cohort of 35 American APECED patients, 23 different clinical manifestations were documented, with a mean of 9 per patient [11]. Patients should be screened for gastrointestinal cancers by endoscopy and by gastric mapping if intestinal metaplasia is found. They should also undergo routine dental exams, given the enamel hypoplasia associated with APECED. It is important to screen for asplenia, which can be identified by Howell-Jolly bodies on a peripheral blood smear. Patients with asplenia should receive the pneumococcal vaccine and be treated with antibiotics for signs of infection. With proper screening and treatment, morbidity is reduced in this patient population.

Outcome

The patient has been treated with calcium and calcitriol with the goal of maintaining calcium in the low-normal range. He continues to have episodes of thrush, which resolve with

2-week courses of fluconazole. He acquired adrenal insufficiency in adolescence with positive 21-hydroxylase antibodies
and is managed with hydrocortisone and fludrocortisone.
Early-onset hypertension, which is reported with APECED,
developed in late adolescence leading to stage 3 chronic kidney disease with glomerulosclerosis and arteriosclerosis. The
patient continues to have fat malabsorption as well as vitamin
B12 deficiency, IgA deficiency, vitiligo, alopecia universalis,
and dystrophic fingernails (Fig. 5.1). In his 30s, he was found
to have intestinal metaplasia of the stomach on endoscopy
and was screened with gastric mapping. The patient is followed by a multidisciplinary team of providers; he is quite
active at work, and he feels well when on his medications.

Clinical Pearls and Pitfalls

- Autoimmune hypoparathyroidism may be isolated,
  associated with other autoimmune disorders, or of
  part of the autoimmune polyendocrinopathy-candidiasis-ectodermal dystrophy (APECED) syndrome,
  which is due to pathogenic variants in the *AIRE*
  gene.
- The clinical diagnosis of APECED is based on two of
  the three components of the classic triad which
  includes hypoparathyroidism, chronic mucocutaneous candidiasis, and adrenal insufficiency or one
  component plus a sibling who has the disease. The
  addition of urticarial eruption, enamel hypoplasia,
  and intestinal malabsorption to the criteria leads to
  earlier diagnosis.
- Hypocalcemic seizures and adrenal crisis can be fatal
  in APECED patients, especially when left
  undiagnosed.
- Patients should be managed by a multidisciplinary
  team who not only address the APECED components that are present but also screen for the development of other manifestations of the syndrome.

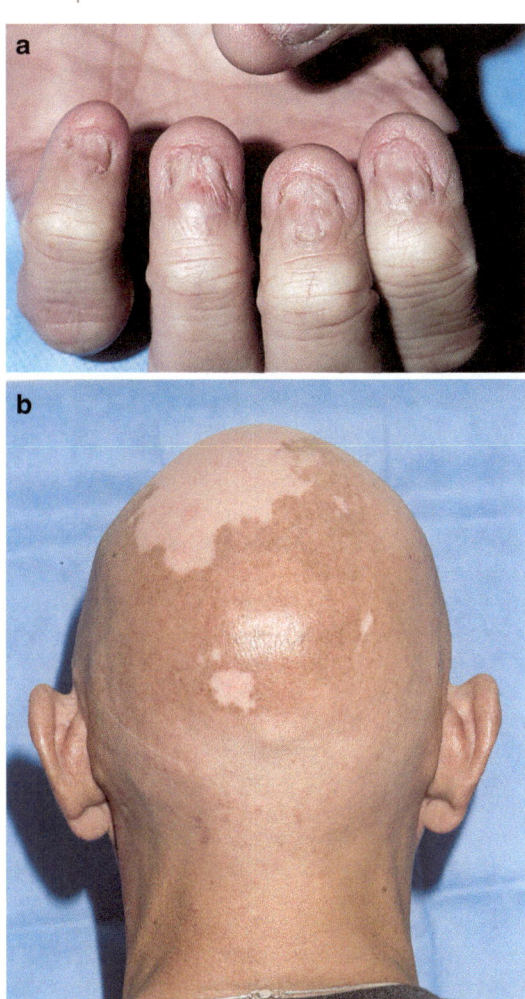

FIGURE 5.1 Skin and nail manifestations of patient with APECED in adulthood. (**a**) Dystrophic fingernails with anonychia and micronychia. (**b**) Alopecia universalis and vitiligo on the scalp. Attempted topical therapies in the past included steroids, pimecrolimus, and tacrolimus without improvement. Sun protection is recommended

Conflict of Interest   The authors declare no conflicts of interest.

Acknowledgments   Work in the authors' laboratory is supported by the Intramural Research Program of the NIH, NIDCR.

References

1. Mannstadt M, Bilezikian JP, Thakker RV, Hannan FM, Clarke BL, Rejnmark L, et al. Hypoparathyroidism. Nat Rev Dis Primers. 2017;3:17055.
2. Goswami R, Brown EM, Kochupillai N, Gupta N, Rani R, Kifor O, et al. Prevalence of calcium sensing receptor autoantibodies in patients with sporadic idiopathic hypoparathyroidism. Eur J Endocrinol. 2004;150(1):9–18.
3. Li Y, Song YH, Rais N, Connor E, Schatz D, Muir A, et al. Autoantibodies to the extracellular domain of the calcium sensing receptor in patients with acquired hypoparathyroidism. J Clin Invest. 1996;97(4):910–4.
4. Kemp EH, Kahaly GJ, Porter JA, Frommer L, Weetman AP. Autoantibodies against the calcium-sensing receptor and cytokines in autoimmune polyglandular syndromes types 2, 3 and 4. Clin Endocrinol. 2018;88(1):139–45.
5. Chamberlin M, Kemp EH, Weetman AP, Khadka B, Brown EM. Immunosuppressive therapy of autoimmune hypoparathyroidism in a patient with activating autoantibodies against the calcium-sensing receptor. Clin Endocrinol. 2019;90(1):214–21.
6. Cianferotti L, Marcucci G, Brandi ML. Causes and pathophysiology of hypoparathyroidism. Best Pract Res Clin Endocrinol Metab. 2018;32(6):909–25.
7. Goswami R, Singh A, Gupta N, Rani R. Presence of strong association of the major histocompatibility complex (MHC) class I allele HLA-A*26:01 with idiopathic hypoparathyroidism. J Clin Endocrinol Metab. 2012;97(9):E1820–4.
8. Anderson MS, Venanzi ES, Klein L, Chen Z, Berzins SP, Turley SJ, et al. Projection of an immunological self shadow within the thymus by the aire protein. Science (New York, NY). 2002;298(5597):1395–401.
9. Fujikado N, Mann AO, Bansal K, Romito KR, Ferre EMN, Rosenzweig SD, et al. Aire inhibits the generation of a perinatal population of interleukin-17A-producing gammadelta T cells to promote immunologic tolerance. Immunity. 2016;45(5):999–1012.

10. Constantine GM, Lionakis MS. Lessons from primary immu-
    nodeficiencies: autoimmune regulator and autoimmune
    polyendocrinopathy-candidiasis-ectodermal dystrophy. Immunol
    Rev. 2019;287(1):103–20.
11. Ferre EM, Rose SR, Rosenzweig SD, Burbelo PD, Romito
    KR, Niemela JE, et al. Redefined clinical features and diag-
    nostic criteria in autoimmune polyendocrinopathy-candidiasis-
    ectodermal dystrophy. JCI Insight. 2016;1(13):e88782.
12. Bruserud O, Oftedal BE, Landegren N, Erichsen MM, Bratland
    E, Lima K, et al. A longitudinal follow-up of autoimmune
    polyendocrine syndrome type 1. J Clin Endocrinol Metab.
    2016;101(8):2975–83.
13. Meloni A, Furcas M, Cetani F, Marcocci C, Falorni A, Perniola R,
    et al. Autoantibodies against type I interferons as an additional
    diagnostic criterion for autoimmune polyendocrine syndrome
    type I. J Clin Endocrinol Metab. 2008;93(11):4389–97.
14. Wolff AS, Sarkadi AK, Marodi L, Karner J, Orlova E, Oftedal
    BE, et al. Anti-cytokine autoantibodies preceding onset of auto-
    immune polyendocrine syndrome type I features in early child-
    hood. J Clin Immunol. 2013;33(8):1341–8.
15. Alimohammadi M, Bjorklund P, Hallgren A, Pontynen N,
    Szinnai G, Shikama N, et al. Autoimmune polyendocrine syn-
    drome type 1 and NALP5, a parathyroid autoantigen. N Engl J
    Med. 2008;358(10):1018–28.
16. Habibullah M, Porter JA, Kluger N, Ranki A, Krohn KJE,
    Brandi ML, et al. Calcium-sensing receptor autoantibodies in
    patients with autoimmune polyendocrine syndrome type 1: epi-
    topes, specificity, functional affinity, IgG subclass, and effects on
    receptor activity. J Immunol. 2018;201(11):3175–83.
17. Kemp EH, Gavalas NG, Krohn KJ, Brown EM, Watson PF,
    Weetman AP. Activating autoantibodies against the calcium-
    sensing receptor detected in two patients with autoimmune
    polyendocrine syndrome type 1. J Clin Endocrinol Metab.
    2009;94(12):4749–56.
18. Eriksson D, Dalin F, Eriksson GN, Landegren N, Bianchi M,
    Hallgren A, et al. Cytokine autoantibody screening in the
    Swedish Addison registry identifies patients with undiagnosed
    APS1. J Clin Endocrinol Metab. 2018;103(1):179–86.
19. Geyer M, Fairchild J, Moore D, Moore L, Henning P, Tham
    E. Recalcitrant hypocalcaemia in autoimmune enteropathy.
    Pediatrics. 2014;134(6):e1720–6.

20. Winer KK, Kelly A, Johns A, Zhang B, Dowdy K, Kim L, et al. Long-term parathyroid hormone 1-34 replacement therapy in children with hypoparathyroidism. J Pediatr. 2018;203:391–9.e1.
21. Linglart A, Rothenbuhler A, Gueorgieva I, Lucchini P, Silve C, Bougneres P. Long-term results of continuous subcutaneous recombinant PTH (1-34) infusion in children with refractory hypoparathyroidism. J Clin Endocrinol Metab. 2011;96(11):3308–12.
22. Feuillan P, Poth M, Reilly W, Bright G, Loriaux DL, Chrousos GP. Ketoconazole treatment of type 1 autoimmune polyglandular syndrome: effects on pituitary-adrenal axis. J Pediatr. 1986;109(2):363–6.

Chapter 6
Syndromic Hypoparathyroidism Due to DiGeorge Syndrome

Bart L. Clarke

Case Presentation

A 44-year-old woman is referred for evaluation and management of DiGeorge syndrome-associated hypoparathyroidism.

Her father was a healthy 26-year-old and her mother a healthy 23-year-old G2, P1–2 female. The patient's family history is unremarkable for hypocalcemia, hypoparathyroidism, DiGeorge syndrome, or other disorders likely to cause hypoparathyroidism. The patient was born at term by normal spontaneous vaginal delivery and weighed 4 pounds, 4 ounces, with her birth length not remembered. She was identified shortly after birth as having a short palate and velopalatine insufficiency. By 3–4 months of age, she was having cyanotic spells. She became listless and developed respiratory failure, requiring cardiopulmonary resuscitation by her father. Evaluation showed her serum total calcium to be decreased at 2.1 mg/dL (normal, 8.5–10.5), with serum phosphorus increased at 10.2 mg/dL (normal, 2.5–4.5). She was diagnosed

B. L. Clarke (✉)
Mayo Clinic, Rochester, MN, USA
e-mail: clarke.bart@mayo.edu

© Springer Nature Switzerland AG 2020
N. E. Cusano (ed.), *Hypoparathyroidism*,
https://doi.org/10.1007/978-3-030-29433-5_6

with hypoparathyroidism, but DiGeorge syndrome was reportedly ruled out initially because of the presence of 10% small lymphocytes on her peripheral blood smear. She was subsequently diagnosed with DiGeorge syndrome by fluorescent in situ hybridization showing a 46,XX karyotype with only a single TUPLE-1 locus on chromosome 22q11.2, indicating a deletion of the DiGeorge/velocardiofacial chromosomal critical region.

She subsequently underwent four surgical repairs of her palate. Her language development was markedly delayed, and she could not speak well until her final palate repair at age 5 years. She had persistent hypernasal speech after surgery and poor school performance due to learning difficulties. She required special education classes. She eventually completed 2 years of college and worked in a manufacturing position. She lives at home and performs her own activities of daily living.

She developed severe hypothyroidism at age 22 years and was started on thyroid hormone replacement. She has been maintained on a stable dose of levothyroxine 137 mcg each day since then. Her past medical history is otherwise significant for mild asthma, eczema, recurrent ear infections, cholecystectomy in March 1996, umbilical hernia repair, an accidental burn on her left shoulder during childhood, and arthroscopic right knee surgery. She has not previously had neck surgery. She does not have cardiac or major vessel abnormalities.

She took PTH(1–34) for 6 years. She initially took PTH(1–34) 20 mcg three times a day and eventually decreased this to twice a day. She noted marked improvement in her overall health during her PTH(1–34) treatment. Even though she had a learning disability in grade school and high school, PTH(1–34) treatment allowed her IQ to increase by 20 points. As a result, she was able to enter college and complete a degree in criminal justice. She then began to study for a degree in psychology. After stopping PTH(1–34), her grades again declined, and she struggled again with learning disability and difficulties with dexterity. She had significant trouble walking and performing normal activities. She occasionally used a walker for ambulation. She finally stopped taking PTH(1–34) due to significant facial rash.

Assessment and Diagnosis

Very few studies have evaluated the prevalence or incidence of genetic forms of hypoparathyroidism. The available studies distinguish postsurgical from nonsurgical causes of chronic hypoparathyroidism, and these give the best indirect estimates of genetic causes of hypoparathyroidism [1–7]. The best prevalence estimate of chronic hypoparathyroidism in the United States is based on analysis of a large health plan claims database, which identified a total of 77,000 cases [1]. About 75% of these cases were postsurgical and 25% nonsurgical. The longitudinal population-based Rochester Epidemiology Project [2] identified 54 cases, with mean age 58 ± 20 years and 71% female, giving a prevalence estimate of 37 per 100,000. In this cohort, hypoparathyroidism was due to familial disorders in 7% and idiopathic in 6%, so potentially 13% of the cohort could have had genetic causes. Other epidemiologic data are summarized in Table 6.1.

Nonsurgical causes of hypoparathyroidism are more difficult to sort out, especially if they are non-syndromic or isolated. Underlying magnesium deficiency or excess or iron or copper overload may be evident by clinical history or ruled out by laboratory testing. Infiltrative disorders, metastatic disease, or prior radiation exposure may be evident from the clinical history. Genetic disorders may be inherited or familial or may be suspected if syndromic features are identified (Table 6.2) [8, 9]. Non-syndromic genetic hypoparathyroidism is often more difficult to diagnose.

Patients with hypoparathyroidism that occurs at a young age and with a family history of hypoparathyroidism must be evaluated for isolated and syndromic causes for their hypoparathyroidism (Fig. 6.1). DiGeorge (velocardiofacial) syndrome (OMIM #188400) is the most widely known syndromic

TABLE 6.1 Epidemiology of hypoparathyroidism

	Number identified/estimated prevalence of hypoparathyroidism	Postsurgical	Nonsurgical
United States [1]	77,000	75%	25%
United States [2]	54|37/100,000	87%	7% familial 6% idiopathic
Denmark [3–5]	2029|24.3/100,000	22/100,000	2.3/100,000
Tayside, Scotland [6]	222|40/100,000	23/100,000	17/100,000
Norway [7]	522|9.4/100,000	6.4/100,000	3.0/100,000 21% autosomal dominant hypocalcemia 17% autoimmune polyendocrine syndrome type 1 15% DiGeorge/22q11 deletion syndrome 44% idiopathic hypoparathyroidism 4% others

TABLE 6.2 Risk of mortality and hospitalization for complications of hypoparathyroidism

	Postsurgical hypoparathyroidism	Nonsurgical hypoparathyroidism
Mortality [8]	HR 0.96 (95% CI, 0.76–1.26)	HR 1.25 (95% CI, 0.90–1.73)
Renal insufficiency [8, 10]	HR 3.10 (95% CI, 1.73–5.55)	HR 6.01 (95% CI, 2.45–14.75)
Renal stones [8, 10]	HR 4.02 (95% CI, 1.54–9.90)	–
Ischemic cardiovascular disease [8, 10]	HR 1.09 (95% CI, 0.83–1.45)	HR 2.01 (95% CI, 1.31–3.09)
Neuropsychiatric disease [9, 10]	HR 1.26 (95% CI, 1.01–1.56)	HR 2.45 (95% CI, 1.78–3.36)
Seizures [9, 10]	HR 3.82 (95% CI, 2.15–6.79)	HR 10.05 (95% CI, 5.39–18.72)
Cataracts [9, 10]	HR 1.17 (95% CI, 0.66–2.09)	HR 4.21 (95% CI, 2.13–8.34)
Upper extremity fractures [9, 10]	HR 0.69 (95% CI, 0.49–0.97)	HR 1.93 (95% CI, 1.31–2.85)

Adapted with permission from Clarke et al. [43]

cause [10, 11]. DiGeorge syndrome is associated with distinctive facial abnormalities, cleft lip and/or palate, conotruncal cardiac anomalies, and mild-to-moderate immune deficiency, as noted in the case description above [11]. Hypocalcemia due to hypoparathyroidism has been reported in 17–60% of affected children [12]. DiGeorge syndrome is estimated to occur in as many as 1:2000–1:3000 births, with the incidence rate of new mutations estimated at 1:4000–1:6000. Because the clinical phenotype varies, findings may be subtle and therefore be overlooked, and mild hypocalcemia may be easily missed. One study showed that in adults with chromosome 22q11.2 deletion, about half were hypocalcemic, with a median age at presentation of 25 years and a maximum age

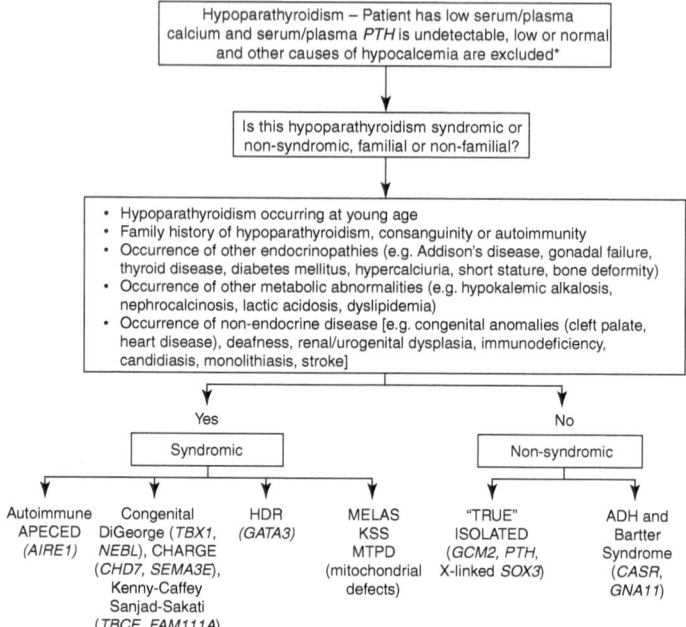

FIGURE 6.1 Clinical approach to establishing the genetic etiology of hypoparathyroidism. The genes for each disorder are indicated in italics. (Adapted with permission from Clarke et al. [43]. Originally from Thakker et al. [44])

of diagnosis of up to 48 years [13]. This disorder may rarely be diagnosed for the first time as late as the mid-60s, with late-onset mild hypocalcemia, and is not infrequently diagnosed in affected parents in their 20s or 30s, after birth of an affected child.

The condition arises from a congenital failure of development of the neural crest derivatives of the third and fourth pharyngeal pouches, with resultant absence or hypoplasia of the parathyroid glands and thymus. Most cases are sporadic, but autosomal dominant inheritance may occur, and unbalanced translocations and deletions in a 250–3000 kb critical region of chromosome 22q11.2 are causative of DiGeorge syndrome type 1. Point mutations have only been found in the

TBX1 gene, and *TBX1* is considered to be the gene causing DiGeorge syndrome type 1, with about 96% of patients having deletion of this gene.

Some patients have late onset of DiGeorge syndrome type 1 and develop symptomatic hypocalcemia in childhood or adolescence with only subtle phenotypic features. These patients also have microdeletions in the 22q11 region, but the reason for the delayed onset is unknown. Deletions of another locus on chromosome 10p have been reported to cause DiGeorge syndrome type 2, with heterozygous deletion of the nebulette (*NEBL*) gene on this chromosome causing the phenotypic features of DiGeorge syndrome.

Syndromic forms of genetic hypoparathyroidism include autosomal dominant hypoparathyroidism associated with bilateral symmetrical sensorineural deafness and renal anomalies including bilateral cysts compressing the glomeruli and renal tubules (HDR), associated with autosomal dominant mutations in the *GATA3* gene on chromosome 10p14–10-pter (OMIM #146255 and OMIM #256340) [14, 15]. The renal anomalies and hearing loss have variable penetrance. Over 90% of patients with two of the three features of the syndrome have a *GATA3* mutation.

Kenny-Caffey syndrome (OMIM #244460) [16] and Sanjad-Sakati syndrome (OMIM #241410) [17] are associated with autosomal recessive hypoparathyroidism, growth and mental retardation, and dysmorphism. Kenny-Caffey syndrome type 1 and Sanjad-Sakati syndrome are due to autosomal dominant or recessive mutations in the tubulin cofactor E (*TBCE*) gene on chromosome 1q42-q43. Kenny-Caffey syndrome type 2 is associated with autosomal recessive *FAM111A* gene mutations on chromosome 11q12.1. Hypoparathyroidism occurs in over 50% of patients with Kenny-Caffey syndrome, which is associated with short stature, osteosclerosis and cortical thickening of long bones, delayed closure of the anterior fontanelle, basal ganglia calcification, nanophthalmos, and hyperopia. Sanjad-Sakati syndrome is associated with hypoparathyroidism, severe growth failure, and dysmorphic features.

The coloboma-heart anomaly-choanal atresia-retardation-genital-ear anomalies (CHARGE) syndrome is due to autosomal dominant mutations of chromodomain helicase DNA-binding protein 7 (*CHD7*), a transcriptional regulator that binds to enhancer elements in the nucleoplasm [18]. These mutations occur on chromosome 8q12.1–12.2. A minority of patients with the CHARGE syndrome may have mutations involving semaphorin 3E (*SEMA3E*) on chromosome 7q21.11 that controls cell positioning during embryonic development [19].

Barakat syndrome is an autosomal recessive disorder associated with hypoparathyroidism and nerve deafness with steroid-resistant nephrosis leading to chronic kidney disease [20], but the causative mutation has not yet been identified. Dubowitz syndrome is an autosomal recessive disorder associated with hypoparathyroidism and intrauterine growth retardation, short stature, microcephaly, mental retardation, eczema, blepharophimosis, ptosis, and micrognathia [21]. The mutation causing this disorder is also not yet identified.

Kearns-Sayre syndrome (OMIM #530000) [22], MELAS syndrome [23], and mitochondrial trifunctional protein dysfunction syndrome (MTPDS) [24] are associated with hypoparathyroidism with metabolic disturbances and congenital anomalies and are associated with rare maternal mitochondrial gene defects. Kearns-Sayre syndrome is associated with progressive external ophthalmoplegia and pigmentary retinopathy before age 20 years and frequently associated with heart block or cardiomyopathy. MELAS syndrome is associated with childhood onset of mitochondrial encephalopathy, lactic acidosis, and stroke-like episodes. Both syndromes may have proximal myopathy, insulin-dependent diabetes mellitus, and hypoparathyroidism. MTPDS is due to abnormal fatty acid oxidation associated with peripheral neuropathy, pigmentary retinopathy, and acute fatty liver in pregnant women who carry an affected fetus. The role of the mitochondrial mutations in the etiology of the hypoparathyroidism associated with these disorders is not yet clear [25].

Blomstrand lethal chondrodysplasia (OMIM #215045) [26] is caused by a homozygous inactivating autosomal recessive mutation in the parathyroid hormone/parathyroid hormone-related peptide receptor. Patients with this disorder typically have hypoparathyroidism with early death, significantly advanced bone maturation, and accelerated chondrocyte differentiation, as well as abnormal breast development and tooth impaction.

A number of other rare genetic mutations may cause hypocalcemia, most often detected in infancy or childhood. The second most common cause of hypoparathyroidism may be constitutively activating calcium-sensing receptor (*CaSR*) mutations causing autosomal dominant hypocalcemia (OMIM #14598) (Chaps. 7 and 9). Destruction of the parathyroid glands by autoantibodies may occur with autoimmune polyglandular syndrome type 1 (APS1), which is an autosomal recessive disorder most commonly appearing in childhood or adolescence, and caused by mutations in the autoimmune regulator (*AIRE*) gene (OMIM #240300 and OMIM #607358) (Chap. 5).

Familial isolated hypoparathyroidism due to autosomal recessive (OMIM #168450.0002) or dominant (OMIM #168450.0001) mutations in the pre–pro*PTH* gene on chromosome 11p15 has been reported [27, 28]. A number of different mutations causing this disorder have been reported from different families. Isolated parathyroid gland dysgenesis due to mutations in a number of critical transcription factors regulating parathyroid gland development such as autosomal recessive or dominant *GCMB* (glial cells missing B) (OMIM #603716), [29–31] *GCM2* (glial cells missing 2) [34] or *GATA3* [20, 21] have been reported. Patients with X-linked recessive Sry-box 3 mutations harbor a deletion from chromosome 2p25 with an insertion near the *SOX3* gene on chromosome Xq26-q27 [34]. This leads to a defect in parathyroid gland development (Table 6.3).

Table 6.3 Genetic disorders associated with hypoparathyroidism

Disease	Inheritance	Gene/protein	Chromosome
Syndromic forms			
APS1	Autosomal recessive	*AIRE-1*	21q22.3
DiGeorge type 1	Autosomal dominant	*TBX1*	22q11.2/10p
DiGeorge type 2	Autosomal dominant	*NEBL*	10p13–p12
CHARGE	Autosomal dominant	*CHD7, SEMA3E*	8q12.1–q12.2, 7q21.11
HDR	Autosomal dominant	*GATA3*	10p14
Kenny-Caffey type 1 Sanjad-Sakati	Autosomal dominant/ recessive	*TBCE*	1q42.3
Kenny-Caffey type 2	Autosomal recessive	*FAM111A*	11q12.1
Barakat	Autosomal recessive[a]	Unknown	?*
Dubowitz	Autosomal recessive[a]	Unknown	?*
Bartter type 5	Autosomal dominant	*CaSR*	3q21.1
Lymphedema	Autosomal recessive	Unknown	?*

	Inheritance	Gene	Location
Nephropathy, nerve deafness	Autosomal dominant[a]	Unknown	?*
Nerve deafness without renal dysplasia	Autosomal dominant	Unknown	?*
KSS, MELAS, MTPDS	Maternal	Mitochondrial genome	
Non-syndromic forms			
Isolated hypoparathyroidism	Autosomal dominant	*PTH, GCMB*	11p15[b], 6p24.2
	Autosomal recessive	*PTH, GCMB*	11p15[b], 6p24.2
	X-linked recessive	*SOX3*[c]	Xq26–27
ADH1	Autosomal dominant	*CaSR*	3q21.1
ADH2	Autosomal dominant	*Gα11*	19p13

Claudin 16 (*CLDN16*), Claudin 19 (*CLDN19*), and transient receptor potential cation channel, subfamily M, member 6 (*TRPM6*) whose mutations are associated with hypomagnesemia and thereby impairment of PTH secretion, are not included. ?*= not defined.

Adapted with permission from Clarke et al. [43]

[a] Most likely inheritance shown, chromosomal location of the mutant gene not known

[b] Mutations of *PTH* gene identified in only some families

[c] Deletion-insertion in possibly regulatory region

Management

Treatment of hypoparathyroidism is designed to improve or eliminate symptoms, reverse skeletal hypermineralization, maintain acceptable serum total and ionized calcium, avoid hypercalciuria, and improve quality of life [35, 36]. This is true for the genetic forms of hypoparathyroidism also, with treatment more complicated when syndromic features are present. The main complication of conventional treatment is hypercalciuria, with 24-hour urine calcium greater than 300 mg, with resulting renal insufficiency, nephrocalcinosis, or nephrolithiasis [35].

Calcilytic compounds may eventually be useful in treatment of *CaSR*-activating mutations [37]. These compounds alter the constitutively activated *CaSR* and stimulate PTH secretion to increase serum calcium.

Once- or twice-daily injections of PTH(1–34) (teriparatide; Forteo; Forsteo) have been used off-label in clinical trials lasting 1–3 years to improve control of serum or urine calcium and phosphorus in hypoparathyroidism [38, 39]. This approach is not approved by the FDA or European Medicines Agency (EMA) for treatment of hypoparathyroidism.

The pivotal 6-month phase III clinical trial with recombinant human (rh) PTH(1–84) (Natpara; Natpar) was reported in 2013 [40], with FDA approval of this agent as an adjunct for treatment of chronic hypoparathyroidism in January 2015. The EMA gave similar approval in April 2017. Several guidelines for treatment of chronic hypoparathyroidism with conventional therapy and adjunctive use of rhPTH(1–84) have been published [35, 36].

Other investigations of long-acting PTH, other PTH analogs, and small molecule agonists of the PTH/PTH related peptide (PTHrP) receptor 1 are beginning or already underway. Two studies reported on patients who had received previous or simultaneous renal transplants who received parathyroid allograft transplants [41, 42]. Advances in stem cell technology may eventually permit induced pluripotent cells or stem cells to be used to create new parathyroid glands in patients where these did not develop or were removed.

Outcome

After discontinuation of PTH(1–34), she required calcium 500 mg 16 tablets per day and calcitriol 0.5 mg 3 tablets a day. With this regimen, she had frequent tingling paresthesias. She subsequently started rhPTH(1–84) 50 mcg once a day in April 2015. rhPTH(1–84) has allowed stabilization of her serum calcium and minimized a number of her symptoms. The patient takes calcium citrate + D 600 mg/400 IU one tablet four times a day but has occasional nausea and vomiting on this.

Clinical Pearls and Pitfalls

- Chronic hypoparathyroidism due to DiGeorge syndrome or other genetic causes is usually diagnosed in infancy or childhood but occasionally in young adulthood and rarely in later life. Some patients die early of comorbidities, but others survive successfully into adulthood and must be cared for by adult endocrinologists.
- Recognizing and understanding the genetic cause of the patient's chronic hypoparathyroidism is critical to treating the patient effectively.
- Genetic testing is increasingly available to evaluate patients with isolated or syndromic hypoparathyroidism. Making the diagnosis allows for evaluation of associated complications. Clarification of the genetic cause of hypoparathyroidism allows for better treatment of these rare patients.

Conflict of Interest The author declares no conflicts of interest.

References

1. Powers J, Joy K, Ruscio A, Lagast H. Prevalence and incidence of hypoparathyroidism in the USA using a large claims database. J Bone Miner Res. 2013;28:2570–6.
2. Clarke BL, Leibson C, Emerson J, Ransom JE, Lagast H. Co-morbid medical conditions associated with prevalent hypoparathyroidism: a population-based study. J Bone Miner Res. 2011;26:S182 (Abstract SA1070)
3. Underbjerg L, Sikjaer T, Mosekilde L, Rejnmark L. Cardiovascular and renal complications to postsurgical hypoparathyroidism: a Danish nationwide controlled historic follow-up study. J Bone Miner Res. 2013;28:2277–85.
4. Underbjerg L, Sikjaer T, Mosekilde L, Rejnmark L. Post-surgical hypoparathyroidism – risk of fractures, psychiatric diseases, cancer, cataract, and infections. J Bone Miner Res. 2014;29:2504–10.
5. Underbjerg L, Sikjaer T, Mosekilde L, Rejnmark L. The epidemiology of non-surgical hypoparathyroidism in Denmark: a nationwide case finding study. J Bone Miner Res. 2015;30:1738–44.
6. Vadiveloo T, Donnan PT, Leese GP. A population-based study of the epidemiology of chronic hypoparathyroidism. J Bone Miner Res. 2018;33:478–85.
7. Astor MC, Løvås K, Debowska A, Eriksen EF, Evang JA, Fossum C, Fougner KJ, Holte SE, Lima K, Moe RB, Myhre AG, Kemp EH, Nedrebø BG, Svartberg J, Husebye ES. Epidemiology and health-related quality of life in hypoparathyroidism in Norway. J Clin Endocrinol Metab. 2016;101:3045–53.
8. Gordon RJ, Levine MA. Genetic disorders of parathyroid development and function. Endocrinol Metab Clin N Am. 2018;47:809–23.
9. Cianferotti L, Marcucci G, Brandi ML. Causes and pathophysiology of hypoparathyroidism. Best Pract Res Clin Endocrinol Metab. 2018;32:909–25.
10. McDonald-McGinn DM, Sullivan KE, Marino B, Philip N, Swillen A, Vorstman JA, Zackai EH, Emanuel BS, Vermeesch JR, Morrow BE, Scambler PJ, Bassett AS. 22q11.2 deletion syndrome. Nat Rev Dis Primers. 2015;1:15071.
11. Merscher S, Funke B, Epstein JA, Heyer J, Puech A, Lu MM, Xavier RJ, Demay MB, Russell RG, Factor S, Tokooya K, Jore BS, Lopez M, Pandita RK, Lia M, Carrion D, Xu H, Schorle H, Kobler JB, Scambler P, Wynshaw-Boris A, Skoultchi AI,

Morrow BE, Kucherlapati R. TBX1 is responsible for cardio-vascular defects in velo-cardio-facial/DiGeorge syndrome. Cell. 2001;104:619–29.

12. McDonald-McGinn DM, Sullivan KE. Chromosome 22q11.2 deletion syndrome (DiGeorge syndrome/velocardiofacial syndrome). Medicine (Baltimore). 2011;90:1–18.

13. Bassett AS, Chow EW, Husted J, Weksberg R, Caluseriu O, Webb GD, Gatzoulis MA. Clinical features of 78 adults with 22q11 deletion syndrome. Am J Med Genet A. 2005;138:307–13.

14. Van Esch H, Groenen P, Nesbit MA, Schuffenhauer S, Lichtner P, Vanderlinden G, Harding B, Beetz R, Bilous RW, Holdaway I, Shaw NJ, Fryns JP, Van de Ven W, Thakker RV, Devriendt K. GATA3 haplo-insufficiency causes human HDR syndrome. Nature. 2000;406:419–22.

15. Ali A, Christie PT, Grigorieva IV, Harding B, Van Esch H, Ahmed SF, Bitner-Glindzicz M, Blind E, Bloch C, Christin P, Clayton P, Gecz J, Gilbert-Dussardier B, Guillen-Navarro E, Hackett A, Halac I, Hendy GN, Lalloo F, Mache CJ, Mughal Z, Ong AC, Rinat C, Shaw N, Smithson SF, Tolmie J, Weill J, Nesbit MA, Thakker RV. Functional characterization of GATA3 mutations causing the hypoparathyroidism-deafness-renal (HDR) dysplasia syndrome: insight into mechanisms of DNA binding by the GATA3 transcription factor. Hum Mol Genet. 2007;16:265–75.

16. Parvari R, Hershkovitz E, Grossman N, Gorodischer R, Loeys B, Zecic A, Mortier G, Gregory S, Sharony R, Kambouris M, Sakati N, Meyer BF, Al Aqeel AI, Al Humaidan AK, Al Zanhrani F, Al Swaid A, Al Othman J, Diaz GA, Weiner R, Khan KT, Gordon R, Gelb BD, HRD/Autosomal Recessive Kenny-Caffey Syndrome Consortium. Mutation of TBCE causes hypoparathyroidism-retardation-dysmorphism and autosomal recessive Kenny-Caffey syndrome. Nat Genet. 2002;32:448–52.

17. Teebi AS. Hypoparathyroidism, retarded growth and development, and dysmorphism or Sanjad-Sakati syndrome: an Arab disease reminiscent of Kenny-Caffey syndrome. J Med Genet. 2000;37:145.

18. Jyonouchi S, McDonald-McGinn DM, Bale S, Zackai EH, Sullivan KE. CHARGE (coloboma, heart defect, atresia choanae, retarded growth and development, genital hypoplasia, ear anomalies/deafness) syndrome and chromosome 22q11.2 deletion syndrome: a comparison of immunologic and nonimmunologic phenotypic features. Pediatrics. 2009;123:e871–7.

19. Lalani SR, Safiullah AM, Molinari LM, Fernbach SD, Martin DM, Belmont JW. SEMA3E mutation in a patient with CHARGE syndrome. J Med Genet. 2004;41:e94.
20. Barakat AJ, Raygada M, Rennert OM. Barakat syndrome revisited. Am J Med Genet A. 2018;176:1341–8.
21. Innes AM, McInnes BL, Dyment DA. Clinical and genetic heterogeneity in Dubowitz syndrome: implications for diagnosis, management and further research. Am J Med Genet C Semin Med Genet. 2018;178:387–97.
22. Kearns TP, Sayre GP. Retinitis pigmentosa, external ophthalmoplegia, and complete heart block: unusual syndrome with histologic study in one of two cases. AMA Arch Ophthalmol. 1958;60:280–9.
23. Pavlakis SG, Phillips PC, DiMauro S, De Vivo DC, Rowland LP. Mitochondrial myopathy, encephalopathy, lactic acidosis, and strokelike episodes: a distinctive clinical syndrome. Ann Neurol. 1984;16:481–8.
24. Labarthe F, Benoist JF, Brivet M, Vianey-Saban C, Despert F, de Baulny HO. Partial hypoparathyroidism associated with mitochondrial trifunctional protein deficiency. Eur J Pediatr. 2006;165:389–91.
25. Al-Gadi IS, Haas RH, Falk MJ, Goldstein A, McCormack SE. Endocrine disorders in primary mitochondrial disease. J Endocr Soc. 2018;2:361–73.
26. Zhang P, Jobert AS, Couvineau A, Silve C. A homozygous inactivating mutation in the parathyroid hormone/parathyroid hormone-related peptide receptor causing Blomstrand chondrodysplasia. J Clin Endocrinol Metab. 1998;83:3365–8.
27. Parkinson DB, Thakker RV. A donor splice site mutation in the parathyroid hormone gene is associated with autosomal recessive hypoparathyroidism. Nat Genet. 1992;1:149–52.
28. Arnold A, Horst SA, Gardella TJ, Baba H, Levine MA, Kronenberg HM. Mutation of the signal peptide-encoding region of the preproparathyroid hormone gene in familial isolated hypoparathyroidism. J Clin Invest. 1990;86:1084–7.
29. Thomée C, Schubert SW, Parma J, Lê PQ, Hashemolhosseini S, Wegner M, Abramowicz MJ. GCMB mutation in familial isolated hypoparathyroidism with residual secretion of parathyroid hormone. J Clin Endocrinol Metab. 2005;90:2487–92.
30. Ding C, Buckingham B, Levine MA. Familial isolated hypoparathyroidism caused by a mutation in the gene for the transcription factor GCMB. J Clin Invest. 2001;108:1215–20.

31. Gunther T, Chen ZF, Kim J, et al. Genetic ablation of parathyroid glands reveals another source of parathyroid hormone. Nature. 2000;406:199–203.
32. Mannstadt M, Bertrand G, Muresan M, Weryha G, Leheup B, Pulusani SR, Grandchamp B, Jüppner H, Silve C. Dominant negative GCMB mutations cause an autosomal dominant form of hypoparathyroidism. J Clin Endocrinol Metab. 2008;93:3568–76.
33. Baumber L, Tufarelli C, Patel S, King P, Johnson CA, Maher ER, Trembath RC. Identification of a novel mutation disrupting the DNA binding activity of GCM2 in autosomal recessive familial isolated hypoparathyroidism. J Med Genet. 2005;42:443–8.
34. Bowl MR, Nesbit MA, Harding B, Levy E, Jefferson A, Volpi E, Rizzoti K, Lovell-Badge R, Schlessinger D, Whyte MP, Thakker RV. An interstitial deletion-insertion involving chromosomes 2p25.3 and Xq27.1, near SOX3, causes X-linked recessive hypoparathyroidism. J Clin Invest. 2005;115:2822–31.
35. Brandi ML, Bilezikian JP, Shoback D, Bouillon R, Clarke BL, Thakker RV, Khan AA, Potts JT Jr. Management of hypoparathyroidism: summary statement and guidelines. J Clin Endocrinol Metab. 2016;101:2273–83.
36. Bollerslev J, Rejnmark L, Marcocci C, Shoback DM, Sitges-Serra A, van Biesen W, Dekkers OM, European Society of Endocrinology. European Society of Endocrinology Clinical Guideline: treatment of chronic hypoparathyroidism in adults. Eur J Endocrinol. 2015;173:G1–G20.
37. Nemeth EF, Van Wagenen BC, Balandrin MF. Discovery and development of calcimimetic and calcilytic compounds. Prog Med Chem. 2018;57:1–86.
38. Winer KK, Yanovski JA, Cutler GB Jr. Synthetic human parathyroid hormone 1-34 vs calcitriol and calcium in the treatment of hypoparathyroidism. JAMA. 1996;276:631–6.
39. Winer KK, Yanovski JA, Sarani B, Cutler GB. A randomized, cross-over trial of once-daily versus twice-daily parathyroid hormone 1-34 in treatment of hypoparathyroidism. J Clin Endocrinol Metab. 1998;83:3480–6.
40. Mannstadt M, Clarke BL, Vokes T, Brandi ML, Ranganath L, Fraser WD, Lakatos P, Bajnok L, Garceau R, Mosekilde L, Lagast H, Shoback D, Bilezikian JP. Efficacy and safety of recombinant human parathyroid hormone (1-84) in hypoparathyroidism (REPLACE): a double-blind, placebo-controlled, randomised, phase 3 study. Lancet Diab Endocrinol. 2013;1:275–83.

41. Hasse C, Klock G, Schlosser A, Zimmermann UZ, Rothmund M. Parathyroid allotransplantation without immunosuppression. Lancet. 1997;350:1296–7.
42. Tolloczko T, Wozniewicz B, Gorski A, Górski A, Nawrot I, Zawitkowska T, Migaj M. Cultured parathyroid cells allotransplantation without immunosuppression for treatment of intractable hypoparathyroidism. Ann Transplant. 1996;1:51–3.
43. Clarke BL, Brown EM, Collins MT, et al. Epidemiology and diagnosis of hypoparathyroidism. J Clin Endocrinol Metab. 2016;101:2284–99.
44. Thakker RV, Bringhurst FR, Juppner H. Regulation of calcium homeostasis and genetic disorders that affect calcium metabolism. In: DeGroot LJ, Jameson JL, editors. Endocrinology. 7th ed. Philadelphia: Elsevier; 2016. p. 1063–89.

Chapter 7
Autosomal Dominant Hypocalcemia Type 1

Karen K. Winer

Case Presentation

A 6-year-and-8-month-old Caucasian female presented with hypocalcemia and was diagnosed with idiopathic hypoparathyroidism in the newborn period. Hypocalcemia, hyperphosphatemia, and undetectable PTH were incidental findings during a work-up for transient hypoglycemia. During the first week of life, she had both transient hypoglycemia and profound hypocalcemia (6.8 mg/dL) with an undetectable PTH of <2 pg/mL and elevated serum phosphorus. Hypocalcemia was first treated with liquid calcium alone and then a combination of calcitriol and calcium. During the first year of life, she had several urinary tract infections. An ultrasound of her kidney at 3 months old was normal, but at 2 years she had radiographic evidence of nephrocalcinosis with persistent hypercalciuria and below normal serum calcium levels. The treatment regimen included liquid calcitriol (0.16 mcg twice

K. K. Winer (✉)
Eunice Kennedy Shriver National Institute of Child Health and Human Development, NIH, Bethesda, MD, USA
e-mail: winerk@exchange.nih.gov

© Springer Nature Switzerland AG 2020
N. E. Cusano (ed.), *Hypoparathyroidism*,
https://doi.org/10.1007/978-3-030-29433-5_7

daily), hydrochlorothiazide, amiloride, calcium carbonate (250 mg twice daily), potassium (micro-K 8 meq twice daily), a low sodium diet, and macrodantin for urinary tract infection prophylaxis. On this regimen, nephrocalcinosis progressed and she developed nephrolithiasis. Linear growth, at age 4 years, was along the 50th percentile, but a deceleration of linear growth over 2 years resulted in traversing to the 10th percentile for height at age 6 years. There were no gastrointestinal abnormalities and appetite was normal.

Assessment and Diagnosis

Gain-of-function mutations in the calcium-sensing receptor lead to hypoparathyroidism. The calcium-sensing receptor (CaSR) is a G-protein coupled receptor and expressed in the parathyroid glands, kidney, and bone. CaSR binds both calcium and magnesium which induce intracellular signaling. In the kidney, the combined actions of PTH and the CaSR control calcium and magnesium excretion [1–3]. Gain-of-function mutations of the CaSR lead to disordered mineral homeostasis with disproportionate calcium excretion associated with small increases in blood calcium. Patients with this form of hypoparathyroidism, which is also referred to as autosomal dominant hypocalcemia, have intractable hypercalciuria leading to nephrocalcinosis and renal damage which may appear, in the more severe cases, during early childhood. Patients with this disorder were referred to us because of profound hypocalcemia which was unresponsive to high doses of active vitamin D and calcium [4]. We studied 23 patients with an activating mutation of the CaSR who, at their baseline evaluation, had moderate to severe nephrocalcinosis. This case report will describe our 10-year experience treating a child with a known heterozygous de novo activating mutation in the calcium-sensing receptor. The variant c.2495>C had been previously described in association with autosomal dominant hypoparathyroidism (mutational analysis: Athena Diagnostics). The patient was referred at age 6 years old because of failure to thrive and worsening renal function while receiving conventional therapy with calcitriol, calcium, and thiazide diuretics.

Management

After a baseline evaluation lasting 4 days, calcitriol, calcium supplements, hydrochlorothiazide, and amiloride were discontinued, and subcutaneous PTH(1–34) injections and oral magnesium supplements (2400 mg/day divided into three equal doses) were initiated. Initial PTH dose was 7 mcg (0.3 mcg/kg) by subcutaneous injection given twice daily. Height was 111.5 cm (9%); Z-score, −1.32; weight, 21.2 kg (38%); Z-score, −0.31; and body surface area (BSA), 0.8. There was enamel hypoplasia of her teeth. Urine calcium excretion range during baseline evaluation ranged 12.7–23.8 mmol/24 corrected for body surface area. Creatinine clearance was 106 mL/min/1.73 M^2. Computed tomography (CT) of the kidney showed bilateral nephrocalcinosis. The bone age was 5 years and was measured at a chronological age of 6 years and 8 months. The patient was discharged after a week of inpatient observation on 9 mcg (0.4 mcg/kg) PTH(1–34) twice daily. During the first year, with weekly titration, the dose gradually increased to 30 mcg twice daily and subsequently titrated down to 20 mcg twice daily (1.4 mcg/kg/day) PTH(1–34). Over the subsequent 6.5 years, the PTH dose was maintained between 0.3 and 0.7 mcg/kg/day. Magnesium oxide dose was 1600 mg daily.

After 1.5 years of therapy, there were no urinary tract infections, and there was evidence of remarkable catch up growth. The patient's height had increased from baseline stature in the 9th percentile to the 25th percentile. Urine creatinine clearance and serum creatinine levels remained normal. Overall control of hypoparathyroidism had improved with decreased hypocalcemic symptoms and reduced need for acute medical attention. PTH injections continued for 10 years. Mean PTH dose was 0.85 ± 0.9 mcg/kg/day. Serum calcium levels remained mostly below the normal range (average 1.91 mmol/L ± 0.29), and mean serum phosphate 1.93 ± 0.29 mmol/L remained above the normal range. Serum magnesium was below the normal range 0.62 mmol/L with elevated urine magnesium excretion levels 8.35 ± 2.52 mmol/24 h/1.73 BSA. Average urine calcium excretion corrected for body surface area was 7.34 ± 1.94 mmol/24 h/1.73 M^2 (normal: 1.25–7.5 mmol/24 h). Mean alkaline phosphatase (204.65 ± 57.2 U/L, normal: 51–332 U/L) and 25-hydroxyvitamin D levels were normal (43.6 ± 8.18 ng/mL) at baseline and throughout the study.

The patient received twice daily PTH(1–34) during the initial 6 years and then thrice daily injections. Thrice daily (6.5–10 years) compared to twice daily PTH(1–34) (0.5–6 years) injections reduced mean PTH(1–34) dose from 40.2 mcg/day (1.4 mcg/kg/day) to 19.5 mcg/day (0.54 mcg/kg/day, $P < 0.0003$), alkaline phosphatase (from 224 to 154 U/L), and 24-h urine magnesium (all $P < 0.01$), without significant change in 24-h BSA-corrected urine calcium. A 3-month trial of PTH(1–34) given through an insulin pump reduced the total daily dose necessary to maintain normal serum and urine calcium levels by 60% from 0.89 mcg/kg/day to 0.28 mcg/kg/day (twice daily vs pump) and reduced the mean urine calcium into the normal range 5.6 mmol/24 h/1.73 M^2 [5].

At study baseline, ultrasound from the patient's local academic center reported extensive nephrocalcinosis of both kidneys. A baseline renal CT scan, before starting PTH therapy at the National Institutes of Health Clinical Center, revealed moderate nephrocalcinosis, and concurrent renal ultrasound showed severe calcinosis with renal cysts and stones. Six years later, a repeat renal CT had evidence of severe nephrocalcinosis. Renal ultrasounds 2 and 4 years later (8 and 10 years of PTH therapy) both revealed severe nephrocalcinosis. Kidney function as measured by creatinine clearance remained within the normal range. Serum creatinine at baseline was 0.4–0.6 (age 6 years) and 10 years later 0.87–0.93 (age 16 years).

During the 2 years prior to the initiation of PTH injections, linear growth had been deficient. The patient experienced frequent bouts of tetany, requiring emergency medical attention during most episodes of acute illness which led to inter-mittent reduction in calcium levels. Progressive nephrocalcinosis with frequent urinary tract infections emerged out of an attempt to normalize serum calcium with conventional therapy which increased urine calcium excretion levels. Rapid IV calcium infusions given to such patients to alleviate symptoms of hypocalcemia may lead to further kidney damage. Additionally, thiazide diuretics are associated with a rise in urinary magnesium and decreased serum magnesium levels. Excessive magnesium excretion contributes further to the kidney damage. An improvement in linear growth was apparent soon after the initiation of PTH and discontinuing conventional therapy. Symptoms diminished, and the patient reported feeling energetic and performed well in school. We observed excellent prepubertal growth (ages 7–10 years), with growth velocities greater than average (see Figure). She experienced normal growth milestones including adrenarche at 9 years old and pubertal onset at 10 years old. Progression through puberty to full maturation was normal. Menarche occurred at 12 years and 2 months, and periods were irregular the first year and then monthly thereafter. After 2.5 years of PTH, linear growth at age 9 years was 10 cm/year. By age 10 years, linear growth was along the 63rd percentile (141.52 cm; $Z = 0.4$). Bone age was consistently 2 years delayed compared to chronological age. At age 11.7 years, her height was in the 76th percentile (154.4 cm; $Z = 0.7$). By age 16 years, she had received 9 years of PTH; her height was in the 90th percentile (see Fig. 7.1). Final height was greater than her predicted adult height (midparental height), 170.9 cm vs 167.2 cm, respectively.

The bone accrual (BMC/aBMD) velocity Z adjusted for height was decreased the first year following the initiation of PTH in all skeletal sites. This reduced velocity was most evident in the distal radius. Subsequently BMC/aBMD velocity-Z adjusted for height velocity was, on average, normal for the remainder of the study. Linear growth velocity Z scores were higher than normal compared to age- matched norms (based on the BMDCS height velocity norms) [6–8].

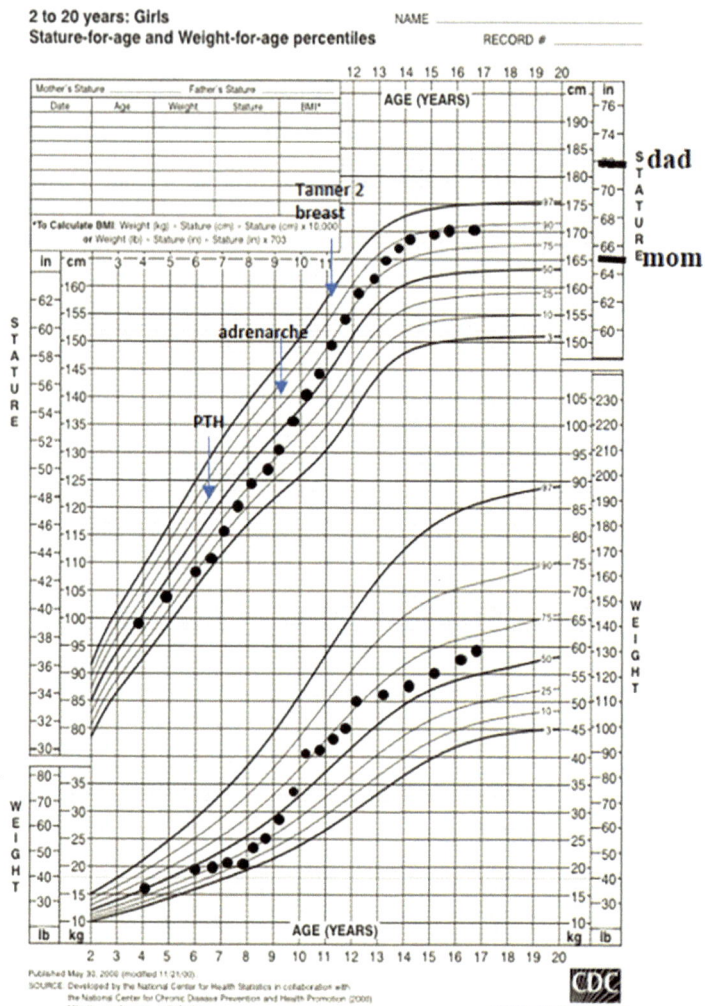

FIGURE. 7.1 Standard Centers for Disease Control and Prevention (CDC) growth percentile curves demonstrating the patient's linear growth and weight gain during 10 years of PTH therapy. Arrows show the initiation of therapy and the time first pubertal changes were observed

Outcome

PTH(1–34) therapy by subcutaneous injection was associated with a clinical improvement including a remarkable improvement in linear growth. Over 10 years of PTH(1–34) therapy, height percentile increased from the 9th to the 90th percentile.

There was an acceleration in growth rate while IGF-1 levels remained normal for age. Urine calcium levels remained at the upper normal or just above the normal range while receiving twice daily PTH injections. Three times daily PTH injections substantially reduced the PTH dose, urine magnesium, and alkaline phosphatase levels. Urine calcium excretion levels, however, were not consistently normalized. PTH delivered through an insulin pump led to consistent normalization of urine calcium excretion and markers of bone turnover. The creatinine clearance and serum creatinine levels remained normal during the 10-year study period.

This case of severe hypoparathyroidism in a child with a sporadic activating mutation in the CaSR illustrates the overall benefit of PTH replacement therapy in a child who developed failure to thrive, nephrocalcinosis, nephrolithiasis, and recurrent urinary tract infections while receiving conventional therapy for treatment of hypoparathyroidism and led to her referral for further evaluation and therapy at age 6 years. Despite excellent subspecialty care from a pediatric endocrinologist and nephrologist and early diagnosis during the neonatal period, control of mineral homeostasis was never achieved in infancy and early childhood. She received treatment with calcitriol, supplemental calcium, thiazides, low sodium diet, amiloride, and potassium supplements. Worsening of renal involvement and poor growth prompted the referral for treatment with replacement PTH. At baseline, nephrocalcinosis was confirmed with both CT and ultrasound.

Synthetic human parathyroid hormone PTH(1–34) therapy improved clinical status, but reducing urine calcium to normal levels remained a challenge. In an effort achieve normal mineral homeostasis, she was placed first on twice daily then thrice daily injection and finally received PTH delivered by pump which finally led to the normalization of serum and urine calcium [4, 5].

This case was one of nine children with a CaSR mutation referred to us for PTH(1–34) treatment [4]. All patients who participated in the study who had imaging prior to baseline or at study baseline had nephrocalcinosis and normal kidney function. Linear growth and bone accrual velocities were overall normal during PTH replacement therapy. Because of their molecular defect and the exaggerated tendency to calcium wasting, patients with CaSR mutations did not generally achieve normal calcium homeostasis with bolus injection therapy [4]. Large serum calcium excursions immediately after the injection led to transient elevations in urine calcium excretion. Prior studies show improvements in mineral homeostasis with increasing frequency of injections and decreasing PTH doses in hypoparathyroid patients of all etiologies and steady state, with normal mineral balance achieved with PTH delivery by insulin pump [5, 9, 10].

Clinical Pearls and Pitfalls

- Activating mutations in the calcium-sensing receptor lead to profound hypocalcemia and disproportionately high urine calcium excretion and a high risk of renal calcification when treated with conventional therapy.
- PTH replacement is the therapy of choice for this disease and must be titrated to normalize both serum and urine calcium excretion levels.
- Increasing the frequency of PTH injections substantially reduced the amount of total daily PTH necessary to maintain normal calcium homeostasis.
- Pump therapy is the most effective mode of PTH delivery as this therapy normalizes serum and urine calcium excretion levels.

Conflict of Interest   The authors declare no conflicts of interest.

References

1. Brown EM, Herbert SC, Riccardi D, Geibel JP. The calcium-sensing receptor. In: Alpern R, Caplan M, Moe OW, editors. Seldin and Geibisch's the kidney, vol. 2. 5th ed. New York: Academic Press; 2013. p. 2187–224.
2. Hannan FM, Kallay E, Chang W, Brandi ML, Thakker RV. The calcium-sensing receptor in physiology and calcitropic and non-calcitropic diseases. Nat Rev Endocrinol. 2018;15(1):33–51.
3. Mannstadt M, Bilezikian JP, Thakker RV, Clarke BL, Rejnmark L, Mitchell DM, Vokes TJ, Winer KK, Shoback DM. Hypoparathyroidism. Nat Rev Dis Primers. 2017;3:17055.
4. Winer KK, Kelly A, Johns A, Zhang B, Dowdy K, Kim L, Reynolds JC, Albert PS, Cutler GB. Long-term parathyroid hormone 1-34 replacement therapy in 14 children with hypoparathyroidism. J Pediatr. 2018;203:391–9.
5. Winer KK, Fulton K, Albert PS, Cutler GB. Effects of pump versus twice-daily injection delivery of synthetic parathyroid hormone 1-34 in children with severe congenital hypoparathyroidism. J Pediatr. 2014;165(3):556–63.
6. McCormack SE, Cousminer DL, Chesi A, Mitchell JA, Roy SM, et al. Association between linear growth and bone accrual in a diverse cohort of children and adolescents. JAMA Pediatr. 2017;171(9).
7. Kelly A, Shults J, Mostoufi-Moab S, McCormack SE, Stallings VA, Schall JI, Kalkwarf HJ, et al. Pediatric bone mineral accrual z-score calculation equations and their application in childhood disease. J Bone Mineral Res. 2019;34(1):195–203.
8. Kelly A, Winer KK, Kalkwarf HJ, Oberfield S, Lappe JM, Gilsanz V, Zemel BS. Age-based reference ranges for annual height velocity in u.s. children. J Clin Endo Metab. 2014;99:2104–12.
9. Winer KK, Zhang B, Shrader JA, Smith M, Albert PS, Cutler GB. Synthetic human parathyroid hormone 1-34 replacement therapy: a randomized crossover trial comparing pump versus injections in the treatment of chronic hypoparathyroidism. J Clin Endocrinol Metab. 2012;97(2):391–9.
10. Winer KK, Yanovski JA, Sarani B, Cutler GBA. Randomized crossover trial of once daily versus twice daily parathyroid hormone in the treatment of hypoparathyroidism. J Clin Endocrinol Metab. 1998;83:3480–6.

Chapter 8
Idiopathic Hypoparathyroidism

Steven Ing

Case Presentation

A 63-year-old man comes to establish care after his prior endocrinologist relocated. In his late 20s, he presented with muscle cramping and spasms of the hand and calves which became daily and awakened him from sleep. About 5 years later, he was found to have decreased calcium and PTH levels and diagnosed with idiopathic hypoparathyroidism. He received conventional treatment of hypoparathyroidism for the past ~3 decades. At his initial visit, he denied hypocalcemic symptoms such as numbness, paresthesia, muscle cramping, fatigue, irritability, weakness, myalgia, mental lethargy, concentration difficulties, anxiety, or depression. His hypoparathyroidism regimen included calcium (as carbonate) 500 mg 1 tablet at breakfast, 2 at lunch, 2 at dinner, and 2 at bedtime, calcitriol 0.25 mcg 1 capsule twice daily, vitamin D

S. Ing (✉)
Division of Endocrinology, Diabetes, & Metabolism,
Department of Internal Medicine, Ohio State University Wexner Medical Center, Columbus, OH, USA
e-mail: Steven.Ing@osumc.edu

© Springer Nature Switzerland AG 2020   73
N. E. Cusano (ed.), *Hypoparathyroidism*,
https://doi.org/10.1007/978-3-030-29433-5_8

5000 IU daily, and magnesium 64 mg 4 tablets daily. His diet included milk 2 cups daily, Greek yogurt 4 oz. daily, and cheese 3 oz. daily. His past medical history included primary sclerosing cholangitis (age 36), Crohn's disease, status post colectomy with S-pouch (at age 39), primary hypothyroidism onset in his 40s with elevated thyroid peroxidase antibodies, pulmonary embolism, and hearing loss. A neurologist recently prescribed glucocorticoid therapy for encephalopathy with improvement, for which he was given a diagnosis of "Hashimoto's encephalopathy." Other medications included levothyroxine (taken 3–4 hours prior to first dose of calcium), digestive enzymes, mesalamine enema, ursodiol, cyanocobalamin, warfarin, bupropion, and duloxetine. There was no known family history of hypocalcemia or hypoparathyroidism including his five children, but his father and paternal uncle both had type 1 diabetes mellitus. On physical examination, he stood 5' 10" tall and weighed 193 pounds; Chvostek sign was absent, and hearing aids and cataracts were present bilaterally. There was no evidence of thrush, dystrophic nails, vitiligo, or alopecia. Laboratory tests showed calcium 9.2 mg/dl (reference range 8.6–10.5), phosphate 3.5 mg/dl (2.2–4.6), magnesium 1.6 mg/dl (1.6–2.6), creatinine 1.06 mg/dl (0.70–1.30), 25-hydroxyvitamin D 40.2 ng/ml (30–100), intact PTH <6.3 pg/ml (14.0–72.0), TSH 0.650 uIU/ml (0.550–4.780), free T4 1.36 (0.89–1.76), urinary calcium 185 mg/24 h (50–300).

Assessment and Diagnosis

Although this patient demonstrated a normal serum calcium concentration, he took significant calcium supplementation, totaling 4 g daily in addition to dietary sources of calcium greater than 1300 mg daily. A review of laboratory tests showed isolated incidents of hypocalcemia. The PTH concentration was undetectable. As patients may reestablish with a new endocrinologist from time to time, the finding of eucalcemia in the setting of supplementation is fairly common. PTH was measured as prior results were not available, but this may not be necessary in a patient with well-established hypoparathyroidism. He was fairly well controlled, but differential diagnosis was a question.

Before concluding a diagnosis of idiopathic hypoparathyroidism, a review of the possible causes of hypoparathyroidism should be undertaken (see Table 8.1, [1, 2]). This patient had no prior neck surgery to implicate postsurgical hypoparathyroidism, the most common cause of hypoparathyroidism.

After presentation with hypoparathyroidism, a few years later, he was diagnosed with primary sclerosing cholangitis, Crohn's disease, and primary hypothyroidism due to

TABLE 8.1 Classification of hypoparathyroidism

Postsurgical 75%
Medical 25%
Autoimmune (*AIRE* autoimmune polyglandular syndrome type 1 versus isolated)
Hypo/hypermagnesemia
Infiltration (tumor, iron, copper)
Radioactive iodine (rare)
Genetic
Syndromic hypoparathyroidism:
22q11 deletion
Hypoparathyroidism-deafness-renal dysplasia (HDR) syndrome (*GATA3*)
CHARGE syndrome (*CHD7, SEMA3E*)
Kenny-Caffey, Sanjad-Sakati (*TBCE, FAM111A*)
Kearns-Sayre, MELAS, MTPDS (mitochondrial genes)
Idiopathic/isolated hypoparathyroidism:
Autosomal dominant hypocalcemia type 1 (*CASR*)
Autosomal dominant hypocalcemia type 2 (*GNA11*)
GCM2
PTH
SOX3

Hashimoto's. With other autoimmune conditions, including one other autoimmune endocrinopathy, an autoimmune mechanism is considered. Hypoparathyroidism is commonly the first endocrine manifestation in autoimmune polyglandular syndrome type 1 (APS1) and typically in childhood. APS1 commonly includes autoimmune adrenal insufficiency and primary hypogonadism. Primary hypothyroidism and type 1 diabetes are less common. His serum cortisol level showed a normal response to cosyntropin stimulation, and 21-hydroxylase antibody was negative. His testosterone levels were in the eugonadal range. Serum glucose was generally normal; hemoglobin A1c and GAD65 antibody levels were non-elevated. Serum B12 levels have been normal on B12 supplementation.

A review of chemistries showed intermittent hypomagnesemia perhaps related to his history of gastrointestinal disorders, but he generally showed eucalcemia and low PTH despite a pattern of eumagnesemia on regular magnesium supplementation. Infiltrative diseases such as hemochromatosis, Wilson's disease, granulomatous diseases, and metastatic carcinoma leading to hypoparathyroidism are rare and not supported by the overall clinical picture as well as normal iron studies and ceruloplasmin levels (and lack of metal deposition on liver biopsy). Radioactive iodine-associated hypoparathyroidism is also rare and was ruled out by history. "Idiopathic hypoparathyroidism" has traditionally fallen within the nonsyndromic versus isolated causes of hypoparathyroidism. Syndromic forms of hypoparathyroidism were considered. He did not show congenital manifestations of DiGeorge (22q11.2 deletion) syndrome such as cleft palate, history of recurrent infections, conotruncal anomaly on prior echocardiography, or developmental delay. Although he had bilateral hearing loss, hypoparathyroidism in hypoparathyroidism-deafness-renal dysgenesis (HDR) syndrome is congenital; moreover, prior tests did not show renal manifestations such as chronic kidney disease, proteinuria, renal cysts, dysplasia, hypoplasia, or aplasia seen in HDR syndrome. Normal height rules out very rare syndromes which include short stature and typically present in childhood such as CHARGE (coloboma, heart defects, atresia choanae, growth retardation, genital abnormalities, ear abnormalities), Kenny-Caffey (dwarfism), and Sanjad-Sakati (growth and severe mental retardation, dysmorphism) syndromes.

Genetic forms of isolated hypoparathyroidism have been elucidated over the years, including gain-of-function mutations of *CaSR* causing autosomal dominant hypocalcemia (ADH) type 1 (Chap. 7), in which the urinary calcium-creatinine clearance ratio is elevated. This patient's fractional excretion of calcium was normal at 0.011, which did not support this diagnosis. Mutations of G_a11 (α-subunit of G11 signaling protein) give rise to ADH2 (Chap. 8). In addition, patients with heterozygous dominant-negative or homozygous loss-of-function mutations in glial cell missing 2 (*GCM2*) which encodes for a parathyroid-specific transcription factor demonstrate parathyroid agenesis. Mutations of the gene coding for *PTH* may lead to defective processing or secretion of PTH (*PTH*, *SOX3*) or PTH action. Thus forms of isolated hypoparathyroidism may be grouped into (1) abnormal PTH secretion (*CaSR*, G_a11), (2) lack of parathyroid gland development (*GCM2*), and (3) defective *PTH* gene.

Management

Germline mutation testing should be considered in individuals in whom a high suspicion of a genetic etiology such as (1) younger age of onset of hypoparathyroidism; (2) additional endocrinopathies, a family history of hypoparathyroidism; (3) history of consanguinity, or autoimmunity; and (4) close relative of a known carrier harboring a hypoparathyroidism mutation [1]. Blood was sent for an autoimmune panel which was negative including NALP5 [3]. Without history of candidiasis, APS1 was not considered, and *AIRE* was not tested.

Although control of serum calcium was not deemed inadequate, nor did he show renal complications of hypoparathyroidism (hypercalciuria, nephrolithiasis, nephrocalcinosis, reduced renal function), hyperphosphatemia or elevated calcium-phosphate product, or reduced quality of life related to hypoparathyroidism, he did meet criteria to consider use of recombinant hormone rhPTH(1–84) therapy given a large amount of calcium supplementation (>2.5 g daily) and the presence of a gastrointestinal disorder associated with malabsorption [4]. After starting rhPTH(1–84) at the usual dose of 50 mcg daily, he was able wean off calcitriol and supplemental calcium while continuing a good dietary calcium intake. Calcium levels exceeded 10 mg/dl prompting a dose reduction to 25 mcg daily and calcium levels reducing into goal range.

Outcome

His calcium levels have generally ranged 8–9 mg/dl with normal phosphate levels, and he has done well clinically, without nephrolithiasis, nephrocalcinosis, or basal ganglia calcification on imaging tests.

Clinical Pearls and Pitfalls
- After diagnosis of nonsurgical hypoparathyroidism is made, consider whether it is syndromic and/or familial.
- Consider genetic testing and counseling for individuals suspected to have a genetic etiology (e.g., young age, family history of hypoparathyroidism, or autoimmunity).
- Treatment of idiopathic hypoparathyroidism with conventional therapy or PTH replacement follows guidelines for chronic hypoparathyroidism generally.

Conflict of Interest   The authors declare no conflicts of interest.

References

1. Clarke BL, et. al. "Epidemiology and Diagnosis of Hypoparathyroidism" JCEM 2016:101(6): 2284–2299.
2. Shoback DL, et. al "Presentation of Hypoparathyroidism: Etiologies and Clinical Features" JCEM 2016:101(6):2300–2312
3. Alimohammadi M, et. al. "Autoimmune Polyendorine Syndrome Type 1 and NALP5, a Parathyroid Autoantigen" NEJM 2008;358:1018–1028.
4. Brandi ML, et. al. "Management of Hypoparathyroidism: Summary Statement and Guidelines" JCEM 2016;101(6):2273–2283.

Chapter 9
Hypoparathyroidism in Children

Rebecca J. Gordon and Michael A. Levine

Case Presentation

A 1-week-old ex-full-term male presented to the emergency room due to parental concerns regarding "jitteriness." He had been delivered via C-section with a birth weight of 8 lb. and

R. J. Gordon (✉)
Division of Endocrinology and Diabetes and the Center for Bone Health, The Children's Hospital of Philadelphia, Philadelphia, PA, USA

Department of Pediatrics, University of Pennsylvania Perelman School of Medicine, Philadelphia, PA, USA

Division of Endocrinology, Boston Children's Hospital, Harvard Medical School, Boston, MA, USA
e-mail: Rebecca.Gordon@childrens.harvard.edu

M. A. Levine
Division of Endocrinology and Diabetes and the Center for Bone Health, The Children's Hospital of Philadelphia, Philadelphia, PA, USA

Department of Pediatrics, University of Pennsylvania Perelman School of Medicine, Philadelphia, PA, USA

© Springer Nature Switzerland AG 2020
N. E. Cusano (ed.), *Hypoparathyroidism*,
https://doi.org/10.1007/978-3-030-29433-5_9

6 oz. and discharged home at 4 days of life. He was being fed with standard infant formula and was not receiving any vitamin D supplements. Past medical history was significant only for a prenatal exposure to gestational diabetes mellitus, which the mother had managed by dietary changes and an oral hypoglycemic agent (sulfonylurea). In the emergency room, the physical exam was notable for poor feeding, irritability, and mild hypotonia. Laboratory studies revealed a low serum calcium level of 5 mg/dL (reference range for age 7.6–10.4 mg/dL), phosphorus 11.1 mg/dL (4.5–9.0 mg/dL), urinary calcium/creatinine 0.6 mg/mg (mean for age 0.27 mg/mg) [1], magnesium 1.4 mg/dL (1.26–2.1 mg/dL), intact parathyroid hormone (PTH) 3 pg/mL (10–65 pg/mL), 25-hydroxyvitamin D 16 ng/mL (30–50 ng/mL), and 1,25-dihydroxyvitamin D 60 pg/mL (10–72 pg/mL).

The infant was initially treated with intravenous calcium and oral vitamin D3 and a change in infant formula to one with a low phosphorus content, Similac PM 60/40. He was subsequently treated with daily oral calcitriol, and for a brief period of time, he was given the phosphate binder sevelamer. He was discharged on a daily regimen of calcitriol 0.2 mcg twice per day plus 200 mg of elemental calcium three to four times per day. By age 1 year, he had developed hypomagnesemia and mild hypokalemia that responded to daily magnesium supplements. Over the next 6 years, he continued treatment with calcium, calcitriol, magnesium, and vitamin D3 and was monitored regularly. During this time, he had serum calcium levels in the range of 7.5–9.0 mg/dL with normal serum phosphorus levels. However, despite maintaining serum calcium levels at target, he had persistent hypercalciuria and ultimately developed recurrent renal stones that required treatment with lithotripsy.

Assessment and Diagnosis

Hypocalcemia in infancy is usually due to transient disturbances in mineral metabolism and in most cases is accompanied by hyperphosphatemia [2, 3]. In neonates, the entity "early onset hypocalcemia" occurs within the first 3–5 days of life and is usually associated with prematurity, low birth weight, maternal or gestational diabetes, or a difficult delivery and is thought to represent an exaggeration of the normal physiological postnatal rise in calcitonin. PTH levels are usually low or inappropriately normal. By contrast, "late-onset hypocalcemia" generally occurs at 5–10 days of life and most commonly occurs in babies who are fed infant formula, which contains far more phosphorus than breast milk. PTH levels can be low or elevated. Other causes of late-onset hypocalcemia include fetal exposure to maternal hypercalcemia, transient renal resistance to PTH, defective intestinal absorption of calcium, or hypoparathyroidism. Hypomagnesemia, either acquired or inherited [4, 5], can also cause hypocalcemia, either through decreased secretion of or responsiveness to PTH.

In contrast to adults, in whom hypoparathyroidism most often results from prior neck surgery, hypoparathyroidism in pediatric patients is typically genetic (Table 9.1). It is especially important to consider DiGeorge sequence (1:2500 live births) in all newborns and infants with hypoparathyroidism, particularly as significant morbidity is related to several of the features associated with this condition, also termed CATCH22, which include cardiac defects, abnormal facies, thymic aplasia, cleft palate, hypocalcemia, and a 22q11 deletion [6]. The DiGeorge sequence is the most common contiguous gene deletion syndrome, and most of the defects are thought to arise from loss of one copy of the *TBX1* gene [7, 8]. Hypoparathyroidism is usually not permanent, but even in cases where parathyroid function has apparently recovered, there can be recurrent episodes of hypocalcemia during episodes of extreme medical stress [9]. There is significant clinical overlap between DiGeorge sequence and CHARGE (coloboma, heart defects, atresia choanae, retarded growth and development, genital hypoplasia, and ear anomalies/deafness) syndrome, including hypoparathyroidism. Hypocalcemia, attributed to hypoparathyroidism, is more common in CHARGE syndrome newborns (72%) compared with sequence newborns (26%) [10]. Newborns with hypoparathyroidism

TABLE 9.1 Causes of Hypoparathyroidism: genetic and acquired

Disease	Inheritance	Gene	Associated clinical features
Genetic disorders associated with hypoparathyroidism			
Disorders of parathyroid gland formation			
Isolated parathyroid aplasia	AR or AD	GCM2	
	XR	SOX3	
DiGeorge sequence			Thymic hypoplasia with immune deficiency, conotruncal cardiac defects, cleft palate, dysmorphic facies
DiGeorge type 1	Sporadic or AD	TBX1	
DiGeorge type 2	Sporadic or AD	NEBL	
Charge syndrome	Sporadic or AD	CHD7	Cardiac anomalies, cleft palate, renal anomalies, ear abnormalities/deafness, and developmental delay
		SEMA3E	

Hypoparathyroidism, deafness, and renal dysplasia	AD	*GATA3*	Deafness and renal dysplasia
Hypoparathyroidism, retardation, and dysmorphism (also known as Sanjad-Sakati syndrome)	AR	*TBCE*	Growth retardation, developmental delay, dysmorphic facies
Kenny-Caffey syndrome type 1	AR	*TBCE*	Short stature, medullary stenosis, dysmorphic facies, developmental delay
Kenny-Caffey syndrome type 2	AD	*FAM111A*	Similar to type 1, but clinically distinguished by the absence of mental retardation
Mitochondrial diseases	Maternal		
Kearns-Sayre syndrome			Encephalomyopathy, ophthalmoplegia, retinitis pigmentosa, and heart block
Pearson marrow-pancreas syndrome			Pancreatic dysfunction, sideroblastic anemia, neutropenia, and thrombocytopenia
MELAS			Mitochondrial myopathy, encephalopathy, lactic acidosis, and stroke-like episodes

(continued)

TABLE 9.1 (continued)

Disease	Inheritance	Gene	Associated clinical features
LCHAD		*MTP*	
MCADD		*ACADM*	
Disorders of parathyroid hormone synthesis or secretion			
PTH gene mutations	AD or AR	*PTH*	
AD hypocalcemia type 1	AD or sporadic	*CASR*	Hypercalciuria
AD hypocalcemia type 2	AD or sporadic	*GNA11*	Growth retardation
Disorders of parathyroid gland destruction			
Autoimmune polyendocrinopathy-candidiasis-ectodermal dystrophy	AR, AD or sporadic	*AIRE*	Mucocutaneous candidiasis and adrenal insufficiency
Disorders of resistance to parathyroid hormone			
Pseudohypoparathyroidism Ia	AD (maternal)	*GNAS*	Albright hereditary osteodystrophy; multihormone resistance

Pseudopseudohypoparathyroidism	AD (paternal)	GNAS	Albright hereditary osteodystrophy but lacks biochemical hypoparathyroidism
Pseudohypoparathyroidism Ib	AD or sporadic	STX16, NESP55, AS exons	PTH resistance, partial resistance to TSH
Pseudohypoparathyroidism Ic	AD (maternal)	GNAS	Albright hereditary osteodystrophy, multihormone resistance
Acquired causes of hypoparathyroidism	N/A	N/A	
Surgical damage or removal of parathyroids			
Infiltration of parathyroid glands by iron, copper or tumor			
Hypo- and hypermagnesemia			

who fail their hearing test should be suspected of carrying a dominant mutation in *GATA3*, which encodes a transcription factor that is required for normal development of the parathyroid glands, the inner ear, and the kidneys. Patients with *GATA3* mutations may have isolated deafness, or deafness in association with hypoparathyroidism and/or renal anomalies, which is termed the hypoparathyroidism, deafness, and renal dysplasia (HDR) syndrome [11–13].

The most common genetic cause of non-syndromic hypoparathyroidism is an activating mutation in the *CASR* gene encoding the calcium-sensing receptor (CASR) [14]. The CASR is a G protein-coupled receptor which is highly expressed on the surface of the parathyroid cell. This receptor senses the concentration of ionized calcium in the extracellular fluid, and binding of calcium to the CASR leads to generation of intracellular signals in parathyroid cells that reduce synthesis and secretion of PTH. Activating mutations lead to generation of CASRs that amplify calcium-induced signal generation and thereby reduce PTH secretion even when serum calcium levels are normal or low. The CASR is also highly expressed in the kidney, where it has inhibitory effects on the reabsorption of calcium, potassium, sodium, and water depending on the segment of the tubule. Activating mutations of the CASR lead to an increase in the fractional excretion of calcium and, thereby, hypercalciuria. Hypercalciuria is more severe than in other forms of hypoparathyroidism, and calcium may still be detectable in the urine even when serum calcium levels are low. Patients with activating mutations of the *CASR* can also manifest type 5 Bartter syndrome, which can cause hypokalemia and hypomagnesemia.

The young age at which this patient developed hypoparathyroidism and the presence of detectable serum levels of PTH, hypomagnesemia, and persistent hypercalciuria are all most consistent with autosomal dominant hypocalcemia (ADH) type 1, which is due to heterozygous activating mutations in the *CASR* gene encoding the calcium-sensing receptor [15]. In contrast, heterozygous gain-of-function mutations in *GNA11*, which encodes the alpha-subunit of the heterotrimeric G protein, G11, which couples the CASR to intracellular signal generating mechanisms in the parathyroid gland, cause ADH type 2 [16]. ADH2 is associated with less hypercalciuria and greater growth restriction than ADH1 [17]. Remarkably, loss-of-function mutations in the *CASR* [18] and *GNA11* [16] cause the contrasting phenotype of familial hypocalciuric hypercalcemia type 1 and 2, respectively.

Other important genetic causes of isolated hypoparathyroidism include autosomal recessive [19] and dominant [20] mutations in the *PTH* gene, including at least one mutation that leads to production of a biologically inactive PTH molecule [21], but parathyroid tissue is presumably intact in these patients. By contrast, parathyroid glands fail to develop in patients with dominant [22, 23] and recessive [24, 25] mutations of *GCM2*, which encodes a critical parathyroid-specific transcription factor. Loss-of-function mutations lead to accelerated apoptosis of embryonal parathyroid cells and hypoparathyroidism, while gain-of-function *GCM2* mutations are an uncommon cause of familial hyperparathyroidism [26].

It is important to identify the underlying etiology of hypoparathyroidism, especially in pediatric patients, as knowledge of the specific gene involved can alert the clinician to the association of additional syndromic features (e.g., a variety of endocrine defects can occur in patients who have the polyglandular autoimmune syndrome type 1 due to *AIRE* mutations). Identification of a specific genetic defect also facilitates screening of other family members, including some affected subjects who are as yet asymptomatic. Finally, understanding the genetic basis for hypoparathyroidism can provide insights into natural history and broaden appreciation of phenotypic diversity [15, 27]. For example, molecular genetic studies of familial hypoparathyroidism have now disclosed that some *AIRE* mutations [28] and *TBX1* mutations [8] can cause isolated hypoparathyroidism rather than more complex syndromic hypoparathyroidism. Today, the identification of the genetic cause of hypoparathyroidism is best accomplished by utilizing targeted gene panels, which are more cost-effective than analysis of single genes or whole exome sequencing.

Management

Transient newborn hypocalcemia typically responds to supplementation with oral calcium, which acts as a phosphate binder as well as an additional source of absorbable calcium. Nevertheless, in some cases intravenous calcium and/or calcitriol may also be necessary. Neonates and children with severe hypocalcemia can be given an initial bolus of calcium gluconate (100–200 mg/kg/dose, maximum 2 g/dose) over 10–60 minutes. This can be repeated every 6 h as needed, as determined by serum calcium concentrations and patient response. Given the very short circulating half-life of calcium, a continuous infusion of calcium is more effective than repeated bolus injections and certainly preferred as intermittent bolus injections of calcium lead to wide fluctuations in the plasma concentration of calcium. A practical approach is to administer 0.5–3 mg/kg/h of elemental calcium, using a 1-liter solution of 5% dextrose plus 1/4 normal saline containing 100 mls of calcium gluconate (93 mg of elemental calcium), which provides a solution with a calcium concentration of approximately 1 mg/mL. One can titrate the dose (i.e., infusion rate) according to serum calcium concentrations. In neonates, continuous infusion of calcium is preferred to IV bolus doses. It is advisable to perform cardiac monitoring during intravenous infusion of calcium to avoid serious cardiac adverse events.

In lieu of oral calcium supplements, it is often more expedient to replace a standard infant formula with one that contains reduced amounts of phosphorus (e.g., Similac PM 60/40) and add additional calcium to achieve a 4:1 molar ratio of calcium to phosphorus (Table 9.2). Vitamin D deficiency or genetic defects in vitamin D metabolism are unusual causes of hypocalcemia in the newborn. When hypocalcemia persists for more than a few weeks, it is likely that the infant has hypoparathyroidism.

TABLE 9.2 Treatment options for hypoparathyroidism

Management	Therapy
Acute hypocalcemia	1–3 mg/kg/hour of elemental calcium administered as calcium gluconate by continuous intravenous infusion
Chronic hypoparathyroidism	
Transient or infantile	Similac PM 60/40 and supplemental calcium
	Similac PM 60/40 has 11.2 mg calcium and 5.5 mg phosphorus per ounce
	For example, 5 oz. Similac PM 60/40 has 1.4 mmol (56 mg) of calcium and 0.9 mmol (28 mg) of phosphorus (1.6:1 Ca:P ratio)
	Add 2.2 mmol of calcium (88 mg, 220 mg calcium carbonate) to 5 ounces Similac 60/40 to achieve 4:1 Ca:P ratio
Permanent	Oral calcium, elemental: 50 to 100 mg/kg per day given in three to four divided doses with meals
	1,25-dihydroxyvitamin D: 0.25–2.0 µg/day, typically divided twice daily
	Vitamin D, as ergocalciferol or cholecalciferol: supplement to goal >30 ng/mL
	Thiazide, e.g., hydrochlorothiazide: 25–100 mg, typically divided twice daily
Alternative therapy	Teriparatide [PTH(1–34)]: initiate 0.7 µg/kg and uptitrate as needed
	Recombinant human PTH(1–84): initiate with 50 µg daily and uptitrate as needed
	Calcium supplements as needed
	Active vitamin D as needed

Our patient was discovered to have a heterozygous activating mutation of the *CASR*, and screening of his parents revealed that this mutation was de novo. He did not respond adequately to calcium supplementation and a low phosphorus diet when he initially presented with late-onset hypocalcemia, which provided the first indication that he likely had a permanent parathyroid disorder. Conventional treatment of hypoparathyroidism in infants and children is similar to that in adults (Table 9.2) and consists of an activated form of vitamin D (calcitriol or alfacalcidol) plus oral calcium [29]. We also recommend an adequate intake of vitamin D3 (cholecalciferol) to ensure normal circulating levels of 25-hydroxyvitamin D, in order to facilitate potential nonskeletal actions of vitamin D. Oral calcium is given three to four times per day with meals and thereby can reduce absorption of dietary phosphate and provide a consistent pool of intestinal calcium for optimal vitamin D-induced transport. In some cases, hyperphosphatemia will hamper correction of hypocalcemia, and the temporary use of a reduced phosphate diet and/or nonabsorbable phosphate binders such as sevelamer may also be required until serum phosphorus levels have been reduced to normal.

It is important to monitor serum levels of both phosphorus and calcium regularly (e.g., every 3–6 months), as treatment goals are to achieve a serum calcium level between 8 and 9 mg/dL, a normal serum phosphorus level, and a serum calcium-phosphorus product that is less than 55 mg^2/dL^2 [30, 31]. In addition, urinary calcium excretion should also be monitored. Although a 24-h collection is best, random urine calcium measurement can be performed and is expressed in relation to creatinine [32]. A normal reference interval for the urine calcium (mg/dL)/urine creatinine (mg/dL) ratio is <0.14. Values exceeding 0.20 are found in adult patients with hypercalciuria. In children, the calcium/creatinine ratio decreases steadily with time until approximately age 6 years. Remember that pediatric reference ranges for serum and urine calcium and phosphorus are age-dependent [32–34].

In the absence of PTH, the renal threshold for calcium excretion is reduced from the normal serum calcium level of 8 mg/dL [35], and significant hypercalciuria can occur even at normal serum calcium levels. It is also important to note that calcium excretion is heavily influenced by sodium excretion. Low-sodium diets tend to decrease calcium excretion, and vice versa. Because hypercalciuria can cause nephrocalcinosis and nephrolithiasis, patients should undergo renal imaging, preferably by ultrasound, every 1–2 years [30, 31].

Over the next several years, our patient experienced frequent and unpredictable swings in his serum calcium levels and from time to time had hypocalcemia or hypercalcemia, necessitating frequent changes in his calcium and calcitriol dosing, with close monitoring of his serum calcium and phosphorus. He continued to have hypercalciuria, passing gravel and small renal stones, and on one occasion required lithotripsy. He was started on hydrochlorothiazide and a low salt diet, but with minimal reduction in his hypercalciuria and continued production of new renal stones as documented by annual renal ultrasound examinations. He also continued to have hypokalemia and hypomagnesemia and developed polyuria, consistent with *CASR*-associated type 5 Bartter syndrome and required treatment with potassium and magnesium supplementation.

Due to his frequent episodes of hypo- and hypercalcemia, at 10 years of age, the patient was started on recombinant hormone PTH(1–84) [rhPTH(1–84)], initially 25 mcg daily by subcutaneous injection. He was able to reduce his calcitriol dosage, and he was subsequently advanced to 50 mcg per day of rhPTH(1–84) with further decreases in his calcitriol dose and reduced need for oral calcium supplementation. On his current regimen of rhPTH(1–84), he reports fewer symptoms (i.e., decrease in hand pain and cramping), and his serum calcium levels are more stable. He also has experienced a modest reduction in hypercalciuria with a urine calcium/creatinine ratio of 0.3 mg/mg. Although PTH and PTH analogs are not FDA-approved in pediatric patients due to theoretical concerns of osteosarcoma in patients with open growth plates [36], there is growing experience with the use of PTH and

PTH analogs in children with hypoparathyroidism [37–39]. Previous studies of teriparatide [PTH(1–34)] in pediatric patients, either by daily injections [40] or continuous infusion by pump [41–43], have shown very reassuring results with improved control of serum and urinary calcium levels. It is the authors' opinion that PTH and PTH analogs represent an acceptable treatment option for at least some children with hypoparathyroidism who do not respond well to conventional therapy. There does not seem to be a consistent improvement in hypercalciuria in patients with *CASR* mutations treated with PTH therapy, with some studies demonstrating improvement [38, 44], while others do not [45], and rhPTH(1–84) and PTH(1–34) may have different effects [46].

Outcome

The patient was diagnosed with a *CASR* mutation that resulted in ADH1, a form of isolated hypoparathyroidism. Over 10 years of clinical follow-up, he was also diagnosed with type 5 Bartter syndrome, was initially treated with conventional therapy consisting of calcitriol and oral calcium, but was ultimately transitioned to rhPTH(1–84) with more consistent control of his serum calcium concentration, modestly reduced urinary calcium excretion, and improved overall well-being.

Clinical Pearls and Pitfalls

- Hypoparathyroidism in infants and children is usually due to a genetic etiology.
- It is important to monitor for renal complications of hypoparathyroidism and its treatment, including hypercalciuria associated with nephrocalcinosis and nephrolithiasis.
- The use of PTH and PTH analogs may be an option even in children and adolescents who fail to achieve appropriate treatment targets of hypoparathyroidism using conventional therapy.

Conflict of Interest   Dr. Michael A. Levine has served as an advisory board member, research investigator, and consultant for Shire/Takeda.

References

1. Sargent JD, Stukel TA, Kresel J, Klein RZ. Normal values for random urinary calcium to creatinine ratios in infancy. J Pediatr. 1993;123(3):393–7.
2. Tsang RC, Light IJ, Sutherland JM, Kleinman LI. Possible pathogenetic factors in neonatal hypocalcemia of prematurity. The role of gestation, hyperphosphatemia, hypomagnesemia, urinary calcium loss, and parathormone responsiveness. J Pediatr. 1973;82(3):423–9.
3. Hsu SC, Levine MA. Perinatal calcium metabolism: physiology and pathophysiology. Sem Neonatol. 2004;9(1):23–36.
4. Schlingmann KP, Weber S, Peters M, Niemann Nejsum L, Vitzthum H, Klingel K, et al. Hypomagnesemia with secondary hypocalcemia is caused by mutations in TRPM6, a new member of the TRPM gene family. Nat Genet. 2002;31(2):166–70.
5. Fujimura J, Nozu K, Yamamura T, Minamikawa S, Nakanishi K, Horinouchi T, et al. Clinical and genetic characteristics in patients with Gitelman syndrome. Kidney Int Rep. 2019;4(1):119–25.
6. Goldberg R, Motzkin B, Marion R, Scambler PJ, Shprintzen RJ. Velo-cardio-facial syndrome: a review of 120 patients. Am J Med Genet. 1993;45(3):313–9.
7. Greenberg F, Elder FF, Haffner P, Northrup H, Ledbetter DH. Cytogenetic findings in a prospective series of patients with DiGeorge anomaly. Am J Hum Genet. 1988;43(5):605–11.
8. Li D, Gordon CT, Oufadem M, Amiel J, Kanwar HS, Bakay M, et al. Heterozygous mutations in TBX1 as a cause of isolated hypoparathyroidism. J Clin Endocrinol Metab. 2018;103(11):4023–32.
9. Kapadia CR, Kim YE, McDonald-McGinn DM, Zackai EH, Katz LE. Parathyroid hormone reserve in 22q11.2 deletion syndrome. Genet Med. 2008;10(3):224–8.
10. Jyonouchi S, McDonald-McGinn DM, Bale S, Zackai EH, Sullivan KE. CHARGE (coloboma, heart defect, atresia choanae, retarded growth and development, genital hypoplasia, ear anomalies/deafness) syndrome and chromosome 22q11.2 deletion syndrome: a comparison of immunologic and nonimmunologic phenotypic features. Pediatrics. 2009;123(5):e871–7.

94   R. J. Gordon and M. A. Levine

11. Van Esch H, Groenen P, Nesbit MA, Schuffenhauer S, Lichtner P, Vanderlinden G, et al. GATA3 haplo-insufficiency causes human HDR syndrome. Nature. 2000;406(6794):419–22.
12. Muroya K, Hasegawa T, Ito Y, Nagai T, Isotani H, Iwata Y, et al. GATA3 abnormalities and the phenotypic spectrum of HDR syndrome. J Med Genet. 2001;38(6):374–80.
13. Chien WW, Leiding JW, Hsu AP, Zalewski C, King K, Holland SM, et al. Auditory and vestibular phenotypes associated with GATA3 mutation. Otol Neurotol. 2014;35(4):577–81.
14. Pearce SH, Williamson C, Kifor O, Bai M, Coulthard MG, Davies M, et al. A familial syndrome of hypocalcemia with hypercalciuria due to mutations in the calcium-sensing receptor. N Engl J Med. 1996;335(15):1115–22.
15. Gordon RJ, Levine MA. Genetic disorders of parathyroid development and function. Endocrinol Metab Clin N Am. 2018;47(4):809–23.
16. Nesbit MA, Hannan FM, Howles SA, Babinsky VN, Head RA, Cranston T, et al. Mutations affecting G-protein subunit alpha11 in hypercalcemia and hypocalcemia. N Engl J Med. 2013;368(26):2476–86.
17. Li D, Opas EE, Tuluc F, Metzger DL, Hou C, Hakonarson H, et al. Autosomal dominant hypoparathyroidism caused by germline mutation in GNA11: phenotypic and molecular characterization. J Clin Endocrinol Metab. 2014;99(9):E1774–83.
18. Brown EM, Pollak M, Chou YH, Seidman CE, Seidman JG, Hebert SC. The cloning of extracellular Ca(2+)-sensing receptors from parathyroid and kidney: molecular mechanisms of extracellular Ca(2+)-sensing. J Nutr. 1995;125(7 Suppl):1965s–70s.
19. Parkinson DB, Thakker RV. A donor splice site mutation in the parathyroid hormone gene is associated with autosomal recessive hypoparathyroidism. Nat Genet. 1992;1(2):149–52.
20. Arnold A, Horst SA, Gardella TJ, Baba H, Levine MA, Kronenberg HM. Mutation of the signal peptide-encoding region of the preproparathyroid hormone gene in familial isolated hypoparathyroidism. J Clin Invest. 1990;86(4):1084–7.
21. Lee S, Mannstadt M, Guo J, Kim SM, Yi HS, Khatri A, et al. A homozygous [Cys25]PTH(1-84) mutation that impairs PTH/PTHrP receptor activation defines a novel form of hypoparathyroidism. J Bone Miner Res Off J Am Soc Bone Miner Res. 2015;30(10):1803–13.
22. Canaff L, Zhou X, Mosesova I, Cole DE, Hendy GN. Glial cells missing-2 (GCM2) transactivates the calcium-sensing receptor gene: effect of a dominant-negative GCM2 mutant associated

with autosomal dominant hypoparathyroidism. Hum Mutat. 2009;30(1):85–92.

23. Mirczuk SM, Bowl MR, Nesbit MA, Cranston T, Fratter C, Allgrove J, et al. A missense glial cells missing homolog B (GCMB) mutation, Asn502His, causes autosomal dominant hypoparathyroidism. J Clin Endocrinol Metab. 2010;95(7):3512–6.

24. Ding C, Buckingham B, Levine MA. Familial isolated hypoparathyroidism caused by a mutation in the gene for the transcription factor GCMB. J Clin Invest. 2001;108(8):1215–20.

25. Bowl MR, Mirczuk SM, Grigorieva IV, Piret SE, Cranston T, Southam L, et al. Identification and characterization of novel parathyroid-specific transcription factor Glial Cells Missing Homolog B (GCMB) mutations in eight families with autosomal recessive hypoparathyroidism. Hum Mol Genet. 2010;19(10):2028–38.

26. Guan B, Welch JM, Sapp JC, Ling H, Li Y, Johnston JJ, et al. GCM2-activating mutations in familial isolated hyperparathyroidism. Am J Hum Genet. 2016;99(5):1034–44.

27. Shoback DM, Silva BC, Thakker RV, Vokes T, Bouillon R, Bilezikian JP, et al. Presentation of hypoparathyroidism: etiologies and clinical features. J Clin Endocrinol Metabol. 2016;101(6):2300–12.

28. Li D, Streeten EA, Chan A, Lwin W, Tian L, Pellegrino da Silva R, et al. Exome sequencing reveals mutations in AIRE as a cause of isolated hypoparathyroidism. J Clin Endocrinol Metab. 2017;102(5):1726–33.

29. Rubin MR, Cusano NE, Bilezikian JP, Brandi ML, Potts JT Jr, Mannstadt M, et al. Management of hypoparathyroidism: present and future. J Clin Endocrinol Metabol. 2016;101(6):2313–24.

30. Brandi ML, Bilezikian JP, Shoback D, Bouillon R, Clarke BL, Thakker RV, et al. Management of hypoparathyroidism: summary statement and guidelines. J Clin Endocrinol Metab. 2016;101(6):2273–83.

31. Mannstadt M, Bilezikian JP, Thakker RV, Hannan FM, Clarke BL, Rejnmark L, et al. Hypoparathyroidism. Nat Rev Dis Primers. 2017;3:17055.

32. So NP, Osorio AV, Simon SD, Alon US. Normal urinary calcium/creatinine ratios in African-American and Caucasian children. Pediatr Nephrol (Berlin, Germany). 2001;16(2):133–9.

33. Burritt MF, Slockbower JM, Forsman RW, Offord KP, Bergstralh EJ, Smithson WA. Pediatric reference intervals for 19 biologic variables in healthy children. Mayo Clin Proc. 1990;65(3):329–36.

34. Matos V, van Melle G, Boulat O, Markert M, Bachmann C, Guignard JP. Urinary phosphate/creatinine, calcium/creatinine, and magnesium/creatinine ratios in a healthy pediatric population. J Pediatr. 1997;131(2):252–7.
35. Hebert SC, Brown EM, Harris HW. Role of the Ca(2+)-sensing receptor in divalent mineral ion homeostasis. J Exp Biol. 1997;200.(Pt 2:295–302.
36. Rubin MR, Bilezikian JP. Parathyroid hormone as an anabolic skeletal therapy. Drugs. 2005;65(17):2481–98.
37. Winer KK, Sinaii N, Peterson D, Sainz B Jr, Cutler GB Jr. Effects of once versus twice-daily parathyroid hormone 1-34 therapy in children with hypoparathyroidism. J Clin Endocrinol Metab. 2008;93(9):3389–95.
38. Winer KK, Sinaii N, Reynolds J, Peterson D, Dowdy K, Cutler GB Jr. Long-term treatment of 12 children with chronic hypoparathyroidism: a randomized trial comparing synthetic human parathyroid hormone 1-34 versus calcitriol and calcium. J Clin Endocrinol Metab. 2010;95(6):2680–8.
39. Winer KK. Advances in the treatment of hypoparathyroidism with PTH 1-34. Bone. 2019;120:535–41.
40. Peterson D, Cutler GB Jr, Reynolds J, Dowdy K, Sinaii N, Winer KK. Long-term treatment of 12 children with chronic hypoparathyroidism: a randomized trial comparing synthetic human parathyroid hormone 1-34 versus calcitriol and calcium. J Clin Endocrinol Metabol. 2010;95(6):2680–8.
41. Winer KK, Zhang B, Shrader JA, Peterson D, Smith M, Albert PS, et al. Synthetic human parathyroid hormone 1-34 replacement therapy: a randomized crossover trial comparing pump versus injections in the treatment of chronic hypoparathyroidism. J Clin Endocrinol Metab. 2012;97(2):391–9.
42. Winer KK, Fulton KA, Albert PS, Cutler GB. Effects of pump versus twice-daily injection delivery of synthetic parathyroid hormone 1-34 in children with severe congenital hypoparathyroidism. J Pediatr. 2014;165(3):556–63. e1
43. Winer KK, Kelly A, Johns A, Zhang B, Dowdy K, Kim L, et al. Long-term parathyroid hormone 1-34 replacement therapy in children with hypoparathyroidism. J Pediatr. 2018;203:391–9 e1.
44. Burkett L, Mittelman SD, Geffner ME, Hendy GN, Mosesova I, Canaff L, et al. A hypocalcemic child with a novel activating mutation of the calcium-sensing receptor gene: successful treatment with recombinant human parathyroid hormone. J Clin Endocrinol Metabol. 2006;91(7):2474–9.

45. Theman TA, Collins MT, Dempster DW, Zhou H, Reynolds JC, Brahim JS, et al. Clinical vignette: PTH(1–34) replacement therapy in a child with hypoparathyroidism caused by a sporadic calcium receptor mutation. J Bone Miner Res. 2009;24(5):964–73.
46. Ramakrishnan Y, Cocks HC. Impact of recombinant PTH on management of hypoparathyroidism: a systematic review. Eur Arch Otorhinolaryngol. 2016;273(4):827–35.

Chapter 10
Renal Complications in Hypoparathyroidism

Lars Rejnmark

Case Presentation

A 63-year-old man was diagnosed with mild primary hyper-parathyroidism. He had a history of hypertension but was otherwise healthy. As a part of the standard diagnostic work-up, a renal computed tomography (CT)-scan was performed showing no signs of calcifications. A neck scintigraphy showed a cold thyroid nodule in the right thyroid lobe. A fine needle biopsy showed signs of malignancy. The patient had a total thyroidectomy performed with radical removal of a follicular thyroid carcinoma. Following surgery, the patient was diagnosed with postsurgical hypoparathyroidism, as he developed hypocalcemia with low levels of PTH. During the following years, his disease was well managed by treatment with activated vitamin D (alfacalcidol) at a daily dose of 3–4 μg in combination with calcium supplements. Initially he was treated with 800 mg of elemental calcium twice a day,

L. Rejnmark (✉)
Aarhus University Hospital, Department of Endocrinology
and Internal Medicine, Aarhus, Denmark
e-mail: lars.rejnmark@rm.dk

© Springer Nature Switzerland AG 2020   99
N. E. Cusano (ed.), *Hypoparathyroidism*,
https://doi.org/10.1007/978-3-030-29433-5_10

which later on was reduced to 400 mg twice a day. Plasma calcium and creatinine levels were monitored at regular intervals three to four times a year. Plasma calcium levels were maintained in the lower part (or slightly below the lower limit) of the reference interval. Renal function was slightly impaired with an estimated glomerular filtration rate (eGFR) around 60–70 mL/min.

Seven years after acquiring hypoparathyroidism, a rise in creatinine levels was noted. Within a few months, eGFR declined to 30–40 mL/min. The patient reported that he was feeling well, including normal urination and no (macroscopic) hematuria. A CT urography was performed showing bilateral urolithiasis. On the right side, there was a renal stone in the proximal part of ureter measuring 6x11 mm causing obstruction. A renal stone was also found in the middle calyx on the left side measuring 6x7 mm, but this stone did not cause hydronephrosis. The patient was acutely admitted to a hospital for immediate treatment with a double-J ureteric stent. Later, the stone on the right side was removed by laser lithotripsy. Attempts to remove the stone on the left side were unsuccessful. Subsequently, eGFR returned to a level around 60 mL/min.

Diagnosis and Management

Hypoparathyroidism is associated with an increased risk of renal stones, as shown in two studies comparing risk in patients with the background population. In a study from Italy, 90 patients with hypoparathyroidism (suffering from hypoparathyroidism for a mean of 9 years) and 142 matched controls were examined by renal ultrasound. The study showed a much higher prevalence of renal stones in patients (30%) compared to controls (5%), suggesting a significant eightfold higher risk in hypoparathyroidism (hazard ratio [HR] with 95% confidence interval [95% CI]: 8.2; 3.4–19.9) [1]. In a nationwide Danish historic cohort study, based on hospital discharge codes, risk of hospitalization due to renal stones during (median) 8 years of follow-up was four times higher (HR 4.0; 95% CI, 1.6–9.9) in a group of 688 patients with postsurgical hypoparathyroidism compared to three times as many matched controls [2]. A major difference between the two studies is that most of the patients included in the Italian study were asymptomatic with stones detected by renal ultrasound, whereas patients in the Danish study were identified due to hospitalization for renal stone disease. This suggests that the risk of asymptomatic and symptomatic renal stones is eight and four times higher, respectively, in hypoparathyroidism. Of importance, although the relative risk is markedly increased, the absolute risk of being hospitalized due to symptomatic renal stone diseases was only 1.9% during the 8 years of follow-up in the Danish patients with hypoparathyroidism [2].

In a number of additional studies, the prevalence of (mostly asymptomatic) renal stone diseases has been assessed by different scanning modalities, showing variable results. Some studies have shown a prevalence of 8–15% [3, 4]; one study showed a prevalence as high as 40% [5], whereas a prevalence of 25–30% has been reported by most investigators [1, 6–8].

PTH is of importance to renal handling of calcium. Normally, PTH increases renal tubular calcium reabsorption thereby lowering calcium excretion. Accordingly, a renal calcium leak is present in hypoparathyroidism, and hypercalciuria may occur. Only few data are available on the prevalence of hypercalciuria in hypoparathyroidism, and this is further complicated by the use of different definitions. However, defining hypercalciuria as a renal calcium excretion above 300 mg/24 h, a study from Boston, USA, reported a prevalence of 26%, whereas a prevalence as high as ≈50% has been reported in case series from Denmark and Italy [1, 9]. This in contrast to a prevalence of hypercalciuria of 5–10% in the general population [10].

Patients suffering from idiopathic hypercalciuria are known to be at increased risk of renal stones [11]. In hypoparathyroidism, it is generally assumed that an increased renal calcium excretion is of importance to the increased risk of renal stones. However, this has so far only been investigated in a few case series showing no associations between urinary calcium and the presence of renal stones [1].

In addition to a renal calcium leak caused by lack of PTH, renal calcium excretion may be aggravated by a high sodium intake causing a high renal sodium excretion. It is well-known that tubular calcium reabsorption decreases in response to a high renal sodium load [12, 13]. In otherwise healthy individuals, renal calcium excretion increases by approximately 0.6 mmol/24 h for each 100 mmol increment in daily sodium intake [14]. Of interest, the case presented had severe hypercalciuria in his first 24 h urine collection, which coexisted with a very high 24 h renal sodium excretion. Unfortunately, 24 h urine sodium was not measured in the second 24 h urine collection making it impossible to infer whether the normalization of renal calcium excretion was (at least in part) due to a lower sodium excretion. However, during the course of his disease, daily dose of calcium supplements was reduced from initially 1600 mg/day to 800 mg/day, which also may have contributed to the decrease in 24 h urine calcium. Nevertheless, calcium intake is a double-edged sword in terms of risk of renal stones. A high calcium intake increases urinary calcium. On the other hand, calcium binds oxalate in the intestine, and too low calcium intake increases risk of calcium oxalate stones. In the case presented, stone analyses showed that the stone contained calcium oxalate. Unfortunately, 24 h urine oxalate was not measured as a part of the diagnostic work-up.

Several studies have shown an increased risk of renal impairment in hypoparathyroidism. In a Danish controlled historic cohort study, based on hospital discharge codes, the risk of renal insufficiency was three times higher in postsurgical hypoparathyroidism (HR 3.10; 95% CI, 1.73–5.55) and six times higher in nonsurgical hypoparathyroidism (HR 6.01; 95% CI, 2.45–14.75) compared to matched controls. In absolute terms, the prevalence of patients assigned a hospital discharge code of renal insufficiency was in the range of 5–8% [2, 15]. A much higher prevalence of renal insufficiency has been reported in different case series. In a Danish case series including 431 patients with an average age of 41 years, 21% of the patients had renal impairment defined as an eGFR <60 mL/min [16]. An even higher prevalence was reported in a study from Boston including 107 patients, among whom 41% had an eGFF below 60 mL/min. In a multivariate regression model, eGFR was not associated with either urine calcium values or the presence of renal calcification, but a significant association was found between eGFR and age, duration of disease, and proportion of time with relative hypercalcemia [8]. Similarly, the risk of renal disease increased significantly in the Danish case series with episodes of hypercalcemia, as well as with an increase in the calcium-phosphate product and duration of disease [16].

How to Safeguard Renal Health in Hypoparathyroidism

Biochemistry

- Measure plasma creatinine and calcium levels at regular intervals (3–4 times a year).
- Avoid hypercalcemia – aim for low-normal plasma calcium levels.
- Measure 24 h urine calcium once a year/every second year.

Diet

- Aim for a low sodium intake.
- Aim for *normal* calcium intake – similar to the general population (800–1200 mg/day).

Consider renal imaging

- In the case of hypercalciuria or frequent episodes of hypercalcemia.
- If plasma creatinine levels start rising.
- If symptoms of renal stones.

If diagnosed with renal stones

- Recommend a high fluid intake (urine output >2.5 L/d).
- Exclude other metabolic reasons for stone diseases.
- Consider treatment with a thiazide diuretic.
- If stone sized >6–7 mm, consider referral to an urologist for removal.
- Consider renal imaging at regular intervals.

Treatment

Obviously, urinary tract obstruction is harmful to renal health and may cause renal impairment eventually resulting in end-stage renal disease, as well as it may predispose to urinary tract infection. Of importance, the case presented was asymptomatic without classical symptoms of renal stones such as pain, hematuria, etc. His renal stones were discovered due to routine monitoring of plasma creatinine levels showing a deterioration of renal function. This emphasizes the importance of monitoring renal function at regular intervals in hypoparathyroidism [17]. Although firm data are lacking, it seems reasonable to assume an increased risk of renal stones if renal calcium excretion is high, similar to the general population. In order to avoid (reduce) hypercalciuria, treatment should be titrated in such a manner that plasma calcium levels are kept in the lower part of the reference interval, as higher plasma calcium levels are associated with higher urine calcium values and may increase risk of hypercalcemia [8]. Furthermore, renal calcium and sodium excretion are positively associated and it may be beneficial to recommend to patients a diet low in sodium. A high intake of calcium is also associated with an increased renal calcium excretion. Accordingly, it seems reasonable to aim at a daily calcium intake as recommended to the general population, i.e., in the range of 800–1200 mg/day.

Treatment with thiazide diuretics has been shown to lower urinary calcium in patients with (and without) hypoparathyroidism [18–20]. Furthermore, treatment with thiazides has been suggested to reduce the oral calcium dose required to maintain normocalcemia [19]. Of importance, treatment with thiazides should always be combined with a low salt diet. Although data are lacking on the efficacy of thiazides to reduce risk of renal stones in hypoparathyroidism, it seems reasonable to consider this treatment option similar to patients without hypoparathyroidism who are suffering from renal calcium stones [21].

Patients who develop renal stones should be advised a high oral fluid intake to maintain a urine output >2 L/day. Other reasons for renal stones should be excluded, such as hypocitraturia, hyperuricosuria, etc. If a stone has a size >6–7 mm, removal of the stone should be considered, as spontaneous passage of such large stones is unlikely. It seems reasonable to consider renal imaging at regular intervals (yearly/every second year) if renal stones have been diagnosed in order to assure proper treatment if they increase in size/cause obstruction before renal function is impaired as in the case presented.

Outcome

Three years later, another decline in renal function was observed with an eGFR around 30 mL/min. A CT urography revealed a new stone measuring 12x15 mm in the right ureteropelvic junction causing hydronephrosis, whereas the stone earlier detected on the left side was unchanged with no signs of obstruction. Once again, the patient was asymptomatic with no symptoms of nephrolithiasis. The stone on the right side was removed, and creatinine levels decreased, although creatinine levels remained slightly increased compared to levels prior to this second episode of ureteral obstruction with an eGFR in the range of 45–50 mL/min.

Kidney stone analysis showed that the stone was composed of calcium and oxalate. The patient collected a 24 h urine sample twice during the course of his disease. The first time was 4 years after acquiring hypoparathyroidism (prior to the first episode of nephrolithiasis) showing marked hypercalciuria with a 24 h renal calcium excretion of 912 mg (normal <300 mg/24 h), which was accompanied by a high sodium excretion of 280 mmol/24 h (reference ranges 50–150 mmol/24 h). The patient also collected a 24 h urine sample shortly after his second episode of nephrolithiasis, showing a near normalization of urinary calcium (316 mg/24 h).

The 24 h urine sodium was not remeasured, but 24 h urine citrate was normal, suggesting that the recurrence of renal stones was not due to hypocitraturia.

Conflict of Interest   The authors declare no conflicts of interest.

Clinical Pearls and Pitfalls

- Patients with hypoparathyroidism are at increased risk of hypocalciuria, renal stones, and renal impairment.
- Renal function (e.g., plasma creatinine levels) should be measured at regular intervals (e.g., every 3–4 months).
- If hypercalciuria is present consider measures to lower sodium intake.
- If creatinine levels start rising, examine the patient for urinary tract obstruction.

References

1. Meola A, Vignali E, Matrone A, Cetani F, Marcocci C. Efficacy and safety of long-term management of patients with chronic post-surgical hypoparathyroidism. J Endocrinol Invest. 2018;41:1221–6.
2. Underbjerg L, Sikjaer T, Mosekilde L, Rejnmark L. Cardiovascular and renal complications to postsurgical hypoparathyroidism: a Danish nationwide controlled historic follow-up study. J Bone Miner Res. 2013;28:2277–85.
3. Arlt W, Fremerey C, Callies F, Reincke M, Schneider P, Timmermann W, et al. Well-being, mood and calcium homeostasis in patients with hypoparathyroidism receiving standard treatment with calcium and vitamin D. Eur J Endocrinol. 2002;146:215–22.
4. Rubin MR, Dempster DW, Zhou H, Shane E, Nickolas T, Sliney J Jr, et al. Dynamic and structural properties of the skeleton in hypoparathyroidism. J Bone Miner Res. 2008;23:2018–24.
5. Winer KK, Ko CW, Reynolds JC, Dowdy K, Keil M, Peterson D, et al. Long-term treatment of hypoparathyroidism: a random-

ized controlled study comparing parathyroid hormone-(1–34) versus calcitriol and calcium. J Clin Endocrinol Metab. 2003;88:4214–20.

6. Hadker N, Egan J, Sanders J, Lagast H, Clarke B. Understanding the burden of illness associated with hypoparathyroidism reported among patients in the Paradox study. Endocr Pract. 2014;20:671–9.

7. Lopes MP, Kliemann BS, Bini IB, Kulchetscki R, Borsani V, Savi L, et al. Hypoparathyroidism and pseudohypoparathyroidism: etiology, laboratory features and complications. Arch Endocrinol Metab. 2016;60:532–6.

8. Mitchell DM, Regan S, Cooley MR, Lauter KB, Vrla MC, Becker CB, et al. Long-term follow-up of patients with hypoparathyroidism. J Clin Endocrin Metab. 2012;97:4507–14.

9. Sikjaer T, Rejnmark L, Rolighed L, Heickendorff L, Mosekilde L, the hypoparathyroid study group. The effect of adding PTH (1–84) to conventional treatment of hypoparathyroidism – a randomized, placebo controlled study. J Bone Miner Res. 2011;26:2358–70.

10. Vezzoli G, Soldati L, Gambaro G. Update on primary hypercalciuria from a genetic perspective. J Urol. 2008;179:1676–82.

11. Lerolle N, Lantz B, Paillard F, Gattegno B, Flahault A, Ronco P, et al. Risk factors for nephrolithiasis in patients with familial idiopathic hypercalciuria. Am J Med. 2002;113:99–103.

12. Chan EL, Ho CS, MacDonald D, Ho SC, Chan TY, Swaminathan R. Interrelationships between urinary sodium, calcium, hydroxyproline and serum PTH in healthy subjects. Acta Endocrinol (Copenh). 1992;127:242–5.

13. Muldowney FP, Freaney R, Moloney MF. Importance of dietary sodium in the hypercalciuria syndrome. Kidney Int. 1982;22:292–6.

14. Lemann J Jr, Worcester EM, Gray RW. Hypercalciuria and stones. Am J Kidney Dis. 1991;17:386–91.

15. Underbjerg L, Sikjaer T, Mosekilde L, Rejnmark L. The epidemiology of non-surgical hypoparathyroidism in Denmark: a nationwide case finding study. J Bone Miner Res. 2015;30:1738–44.

16. Underbjerg L, Sikjaer T, Rejnmark L. Long-term complications in patients with hypoparathyroidism evaluated by biochemical findings: a case-control study. J Bone Miner Res. 2018;33:822–31.

17. Bollerslev J, Rejnmark L, Marcocci C, Shoback DM, Sitges-Serra A, van Biesen W, et al. European Society of Endocrinology Clinical Guideline: treatment of chronic hypoparathyroidism in adults. Eur J Endocrinol. 2015;173:G1–G20.

108   L. Rejnmark

18. Kurzel RB, Hagen GA. Use of thiazide diuretics to reduce the hypercalciuria of hypoparathyroidism during pregnancy. Am J Perinatol. 1990;7:333–6.
19. Newman GH, Wade M, Hosking DJ. Effect of bendrofluazide on calcium reabsorption in hypoparathyroidism. Eur J Clin Pharmacol. 1984;27:41–6.
20. Ohkawa M, Tokunaga S, Nakashima T, Orito M, Hisazumi H. Thiazide treatment for calcium urolithiasis in patients with idiopathic hypercalciuria. Br J Urol. 1992;69:571–6.
21. Fink HA, Wilt TJ, Eidman KE, Garimella PS, MacDonald R, Rutks IR, et al. Medical management to prevent recurrent nephrolithiasis in adults: a systematic review for an American College of Physicians Clinical Guideline. Ann Intern Med. 2013;158:535–43.

Chapter 11
Hypoparathyroidism and Cataract

Shira B. Eytan and Natalie E. Cusano

Case Presentation

A 25-year-old woman was referred by her neurologist for brain calcifications on magnetic resonance imaging (MRI). She had presented to neurology after a fall resulting in concussion. MRI brain without contrast noted increased signal intensity on the T1-weighted sequences, within the posterior margins of bilateral thalami, putamina, caudate nuclei, and dentate nuclei which were noted as nonspecific but may represent increased deposition of calcium in the structures. She had a history of hypocalcemia diagnosed 5 years prior in her home country treated with calcium supplements but no history of further evaluation. Her regimen at the time of her visit was calcium carbonate 1200 mg twice daily and vitamin D3 2000 IU daily. One year prior she had presented to

S. B. Eytan
Division of Endocrinology, NYU Langone, New York, NY, USA

N. E. Cusano (✉)
Department of Medicine, Division of Endocrinology,
Northwell Health/Lenox Hill Hospital, New York, NY, USA
e-mail: ncusano@northwell.edu

© Springer Nature Switzerland AG 2020
N. E. Cusano (ed.), *Hypoparathyroidism*,
https://doi.org/10.1007/978-3-030-29433-5_11

ophthalmology with blurry vision and was found to have bilateral posterior subcapsular cataracts attributed to sun exposure. She underwent bilateral cataract surgery at age 24. She had no other surgical history. Her family history was unremarkable. She noted intermittent tingling in her fingertips and fatigue but denied history of seizure, fracture, neck surgery or irradiation, oral candidiasis, or family history of autoimmune disease.

Physical examination was unremarkable and negative for mucocutaneous candidiasis, neck scar, vitiligo, fungal infection of the nail beds, or neurologic signs. Laboratory evaluation was notable for calcium 6.3 mg/dL (8.6–10.5 mg/dL), ionized calcium 0.79 mmol/L (1.12–1.32 mmol/L), PTH 4 pg/mL (12–65 pg/mL), 25-hydroxyvitamin D 53.8 ng/mL (30–100 ng/mL), phosphorus 7.4 mg/dL (2.5–4.5 mg/dL), magnesium 1.8 mg/dL (1.6–2.6 mg/dL), and creatinine 0.83 mg/dL (0.4–1.4 mg/dL). PTH antibody was negative. Thyroid function tests and cortisol levels were within the normal range. Renal ultrasound was without evidence of calcification.

Assessment and Diagnosis

The association between hypoparathyroidism and cataract was first described in 1880 [1]. It is postulated that calcium phosphate crystals are deposited in the lens causing cataract in patients with hypoparathyroidism and a high calcium/phosphate product [2]. Cataracts in hypoparathyroidism are typically of the posterior subcapsular type. Pohjola found a 58% prevalence of cataract in 69 patients with nonsurgical hypoparathyroidism [3]. Goswami and colleagues found a 51% prevalence of cataract in nonsurgical disease, correlated to duration of disease and presence of basal ganglia calcification [4]. In the studies from Underbjerg and colleagues, patients with nonsurgical hypoparathyroidism were more likely to develop cataracts than controls (HR 4.21; 95% CI,

2.13–8.34), with a younger age of onset (53 vs. 60 years) [5–7]. There was no difference between patients with postoperative hypoparathyroidism and controls in incidence (HR 1.17; 95% CI 0.66–2.09) or age of onset. In contrast, Vadiveloo and colleagues noted an increased risk of cataract in all patients (HR 2.10; 95% CI 1.30–3.39) [8]. As the data from Underbjerg and Vadiveloo and colleagues are based on hospital discharge codes and not direct clinical examination, their values may be an underrepresentation.

The lens is a biconvex structure that works in conjunction with the cornea to refract light to the retina. The lens can change the focal distance of the eye, termed accommodation, to focus on objects at various distances. The process of accommodation is similar to the focusing of a photographic camera through movement of its lenses. The lens is composed primarily of water and protein, with light typically passing through a clear lens to reach the retina. With aging or other processes, some of the lens proteins may denature or degrade, forming a cataract and resulting in visual impairment. The lens is comprised of three main parts: the lens fibers, the lens epithelium, and the lens capsule. The most common cataract associated with aging is nuclear sclerosis, involving the central or "nuclear" part of the lens. Posterior subcapsular cataracts involve the back of the lens adjacent to the capsule in which the lens sits. They can cause disproportionate symptoms for their size since light becomes more focused toward the back of the lens. Symptoms of cataract include blurry or double vision, faded colors, halos around light, sensitivity to light, and decreased night vision. Patients with posterior subcapsular cataract may complain of glare as their primary symptom. Slit-lamp and ophthalmoscopic examinations are recommended in all patients with hypoparathyroidism who develop symptoms of cataract [9, 10].

Another potential ophthalmologic finding in hypocalcemia of any etiology is papilledema. The pathophysiological mechanism of papilledema in hypocalcemia remains poorly understood. Papilledema may or may not be accompanied by elevated cerebrospinal fluid pressure, and the term "pseudo-papilledema" has also been used in cases of normal cerebrospinal fluid pressure. It has been postulated that hypocalcemia decreases axonal transport, leading to swelling of the axons and optic disc. If present, papilledema improves with resolution of hypocalcemia [11].

Management

Therapy of early cataract can include change in eyeglass prescription, brighter lighting, anti-glare sunglasses, or magnifying lenses. The definitive treatment of cataract is surgical, with removal of the damaged lens and replacement by an artificial lens. Management decisions are made by the ophthalmologist [12]. Saha and colleagues studied 27 patients with idiopathic hypoparathyroidism from the Pohjola cohort undergoing cataract surgery compared to controls. Patients with hypoparathyroidism underwent cataract surgery at a younger age than the control cohort (34 vs. 58 years; p <0.001) and had a higher incidence of posterior capsular opacification after surgery, requiring subsequent laser capsulotomy [13].

Outcome

Titration of medications for hypoparathyroidism led to current doses of calcium citrate 500 mg three times daily, calcitriol 0.5 mcg twice daily, and vitamin D3 3000 IU daily, which resulted in calcium 9.1 mg/dL, phosphorus 3.9 mg/dL, and 25-hydroxyvitamin D 40.4 ng/mL. She reported improvement in energy and the absence of tingling. She has had no evidence of cataract recurrence. She will be followed at least annually by ophthalmology, with prompt management of hyperphosphatemia or an elevated calcium phosphate product if they arise.

Clinical Pitfalls and Peals

- Patients with nonsurgical hypoparathyroidism are at risk for cataract, particularly at younger ages than senile cataract; there are some data that patients with surgical hypoparathyroidism may be at increased risk as well.
- Hypoparathyroid patients are at particular risk for posterior subcapsular cataract.
- Hypoparathyroid patients with complaints of blurry or double vision, faded colors, halos around light, sensitivity to light, glare, and decreased night vision should be referred to an ophthalmologist for slit-lamp examination.
- Definitive treatment of cataract is surgical, and hypoparathyroid patients may have a higher incidence of posterior capsular opacification after surgery.

Conflict of Interest   The authors declare no conflicts of interest.

References

1. Granström KO, Hed R. Idiopathic hypoparathyroidism with cataract and spontaneous hypocalcaemic hypercalciuria. Acta Med Scand. 1965;178(4):417–21.
2. Blake J. Eye signs in idiopathic hypoparathyroidism. Trans Ophthalmol Soc U K. 1976;96:448–51.
3. Pohjola S. Ocular manifestations of idiopathic hypoparathyroidism. Acta Ophthalmol. 1962;40:255–65.
4. Goswami R, Sharma R, Sreenivas V, Gupta N, Ganapathy A, Das S. Prevalence and progression of basal ganglia calcification and its pathogenic mechanism in patients with idiopathic hypoparathyroidism. Clin Endocrinol. 2012;77(2):200–6.
5. Underbjerg L, Sikjaer T, Mosekilde L, Rejnmark L. Postsurgical hypoparathyroidism–risk of fractures, psychiatric diseases, cancer, cataract, and infections. J Bone Miner Res. 2014;29(11):2504–10.

S. B. Eytan and N. E. Cusano

6. Underbjerg L, Sikjaer T, Mosekilde L, Rejnmark L. Cardiovascular and renal complications to postsurgical hypoparathyroidism: a Danish nationwide controlled historic follow-up study. J Bone Miner Res. 2013;28(11):2277–85.

7. Underbjerg L, Sikjaer T, Mosekilde L, Rejnmark L. The epidemiology of nonsurgical hypoparathyroidism in Denmark: a nationwide case finding study. J Bone Miner Res. 2015;30(9):1738–44.

8. Vadiveloo T, Donnan PT, Leese CJ, Abraham KJ, Leese GP. Increased mortality and morbidity in patients with chronic hypoparathyroidism: a population-based study. Clin Endocrinol. 2019;90:285–92.

9. Bollerslev J, Rejnmark L, Marcocci C, Shoback DM, Sitges-Serra A, van Biesen W, Dekkers OM, European Society of Endocrinology. European Society of Endocrinology Clinical Guideline: treatment of chronic hypoparathyroidism in adults. Eur J Endocrinol. 2015;173:G1–20.

10. Brandi ML, Bilezikian JP, Shoback D, Bouillon R, Clarke BL, Thakker RV, Khan AA, Potts JT Jr. Management of hypoparathyroidism: summary statement and guidelines. J Clin Endocrinol Metab. 2016;101:2273–83.

11. McLean C, Lobo R, Brazier DJ. Optic disc involvement in hypocalcaemia with hypoparathyroidism: papilloedema or optic neuropathy? Neuroophthalmology. 1998;20(3):117–24.

12. National Institute for Health and Care Excellence (UK). Cataracts in adults: management. London: National Institute for Health and Care Excellence (UK); 2017.

13. Saha S, Gantyala SP, Aggarwal S, Sreenivas V, Tandon R, Goswami R. Long-term outcome of cataract surgery in patients with idiopathic hypoparathyroidism and its relationship with their calcemic status. J Bone Miner Metab. 2017;35(4):405–11.

Chapter 12
Hypoparathyroidism and Seizure

Barbara C. Silva and Natalie E. Cusano

Case Presentation

A previously healthy 29-year-old woman underwent total thyroidectomy with central lymph node dissection for a 1 cm papillary thyroid carcinoma, with unintentional removal of one parathyroid gland. Postoperatively she developed muscle cramps, spasms, and tingling. Chvostek's and Trousseau's signs were positive. Her physical examination was otherwise

B. C. Silva
Division of Endocrinology, Santa Casa Hospital,
Belo Horizonte, Brazil

Division of Endocrinology, Felicio Rocho Hospital,
Belo Horizonte, Brazil

Department of Medicine, Centro Universitario de Belo Horizonte,
UNIBH, Belo Horizonte, Brazil

N. E. Cusano (✉)
Department of Medicine, Division of Endocrinology,
Northwell Health/Lenox Hill Hospital, New York, NY, USA
e-mail: ncusano@northwell.edu

© Springer Nature Switzerland AG 2020   115
N. E. Cusano (ed.), *Hypoparathyroidism*,
https://doi.org/10.1007/978-3-030-29433-5_12

unremarkable. Her serum total and ionized calcium level were low, and she was treated with intravenous calcium gluconate, oral supplementation of calcium carbonate, and calcitriol. Her symptoms improved, and she was discharged on 1 g of elemental calcium four times daily, 1600 IU of cholecalciferol, 0.75 μg of calcitriol twice daily, and 200 μg of levothyroxine daily.

One year after the neck surgery, the patient presented to the emergency department with a generalized tonic-clonic seizure. Her serum total calcium level was 5.0 mg/dL (reference range 8.3–10.6 mg/dL), albumin 4.4 g/dL, ionized calcium 2.4 mg/dL (reference range 4.5–5.3 mg/dL), PTH 1 pg/mL (reference range 4–58 pg/mL), 25-hydroxyvitamin D 38.3 ng/mL, phosphate 7.2 mg/dL (reference range 2.5–4.5 mg/dL), and magnesium 2.3 mg/dL (reference range 1.3–2.7 mg/dL). Other electrolytes, glucose, TSH, complete blood count, renal function tests, and liver function tests were normal. She was given an intravenous bolus of calcium gluconate (180 mg of elemental calcium), followed by a slower infusion of calcium. Her symptoms improved rapidly, and her serum calcium increased. Computed tomography and magnetic resonance of the brain were normal. No intercurrent illness or gastrointestinal tract disorders that could be associated with malabsorption were identified to explain the inadequate control of her serum calcium concentration. An electroencephalogram (EEG), performed 11 days after the seizure, showed nonspecific abnormalities of diffuse, non-paroxysmal slow waves of low voltage. She was initially prescribed phenytoin during hospital admission. She was discharged on an increased calcitriol dose of 2 μg per day total and the same calcium supplementation of 1 g of elemental calcium four times daily. Phenytoin was discontinued.

In the following 18 months, whereas the patient reported regular use of her medications, she was admitted to the emergency department twice again due to generalized tonic-clonic seizures precipitated by severe hypocalcemia (serum total calcium level of 5.5 mg/dL in one episode and

5.8 mg/dL in the other). Additionally, she had an episode of acute renal colic due to nephrolithiasis. Her serum total calcium was 7.8 mg/dL, phosphate level 5.3 mg/dL, PTH 1 pg/mL, and 25-hydroxyvitamin D 40 ng/mL. Hydrochlorothiazide (25 mg daily) was added to reduce urinary calcium excretion. In addition, her calcium supplementation was changed to calcium citrate (4 g of elemental calcium per day), and calcitriol was reduced to 1.5 μg per day.

Assessment and Diagnosis

This patient had recurrent generalized tonic-clonic seizures precipitated by severe hypocalcemia. The patient had undergone total thyroidectomy and unintentional removal of one parathyroid gland 1 year before she presented with the first episode of seizure. Whereas only one parathyroid gland was removed, the remaining parathyroid tissue must have been damaged during her neck surgery, explaining the severe and persistent postoperative hypoparathyroidism. She presented with inadequate control of her serum calcium despite being prescribed high doses of oral calcium, calcitriol, and vitamin D_3. Measurement of serum 1,25-dihydroxyvitamin D can be considered in situations where compliance is of concern, but serum levels of 1,25-dihydroxyvitamin D were not assessed in this case [1]. Intercurrent illness and gastrointestinal malabsorption were not identified. Her serum calcium level was very low at the time of seizure, confirming hypocalcemia as the cause. Neuroimaging studies were performed, and structural brain abnormalities were absent. No other metabolic disturbances that could have precipitated a convulsive seizure were identified. Individuals with well-known hypoparathyroidism who are noncompliant can present with acute hypocalcemic states with life-threatening manifestations, including seizures.

Generalized tonic-clonic and focal motor seizures have been reported in individuals with hypocalcemia due to hypoparathyroidism, even without frank tetany [1–5]. There is no correlation linking a specific serum calcium level to the seizure threshold or to EEG changes in hypocalcemia. Atypical absence or akinetic seizures have also been reported, although much less frequently [4]. Ionized calcium modulates postsynaptic excitability and the release of mediators from presynaptic terminals. Thus, optimum calcium concentrations in the extracellular space and in the neuron are needed for normal synaptic transmission. Indeed, an increase in calcium concentration in cerebrospinal fluid was shown to have an anticonvulsive effect [6]. In contrast, hypocalcemia appears to induce a state of neuronal irritability in the central nervous system, which is analogous to the membrane instability of the peripheral nerve in hypocalcemic tetany [7]. In a Danish nationwide survey, Underbjerg and colleagues found that patients with postoperative hypoparathyroidism had a 3.8-fold greater risk of hospitalization due to seizures than controls (HR, 3.82; 95% CI, 2.15–6.79) [8]. Similarly, the risk of seizures was tenfold greater in individuals with nonsurgical hypoparathyroidism (HR 10.05, 95% CI 5.39–18.72) [9]. Vadiveloo and colleagues also noted an increased risk of seizures (HR 1.65 [95% CI 1.12–2.44]) in a population-based study from Tayside, Scotland [10]. Metabolic disturbances, including hypocalcemia, were the most common identifiable etiology of seizures in a retrospective analysis of 139 patients with new-onset disease [11].

EEG abnormalities, including spikes and sharp waves associated with bursts of high voltage, paroxysmal slow waves, have been reported when serum calcium is lower than 6.5 mg/dL. EEG alterations are less evident in the setting of mild hypocalcemia and are completely resolved when hypocalcemia is corrected [7]. In the case here reported, the EEG was performed 11 days following the patient's first seizure, when serum calcium was at 7.5 mg/dL. The result showed nonspecific abnormalities of diffuse, non-paroxysmal slow waves of low voltage.

Management

Treatment of patients with hypocalcemia and severe clinical manifestations, such as bronchospasm, laryngospasm, tetany, and seizures, requires intravenous calcium administration (Chap. 1). Oral calcium and active vitamin D should be initiated as soon as possible. Intravenous calcium can be discontinued when an effective regimen of oral calcium and vitamin D has been achieved. The First International Conference on the Management of Hypoparathyroidism has suggested specific situations in which rhPTH(1–84) therapy could be considered (Chap. 5) [12]. This patient would meet multiple of these criteria for rhPTH(1–84) therapy including frequent episodes of significant hypo- and/or hypercalcemia, despite conventional treatment; persistent hyperphosphatemia or calcium x phosphate product above 55 mg^2/dL^2; nephrolithiasis, nephrocalcinosis, or reduced creatinine clearance to lower than 60 mL/min; hypercalciuria and/or other biochemical indices of renal stone risk; and excessive amounts of oral medications required to control symptoms, such as >2.5 g of calcium and/or >1.5 μg of active vitamin D. rhPTH(1–84) is an expensive medication, however, which should be taken into account when this therapy is being considered.

In this case, the patient had episodes of severe hypocalcemia, with three such episodes associated with seizures. The patient was adequately treated with intravenous calcium in the emergency department, and high doses of oral calcium and calcitriol were prescribed. The antiseizure drug phenytoin was prescribed to the patient following her first episode of seizure, but discontinued upon confirmation that the seizure was precipitated by hypocalcemia. In addition to the inadequate control of her serum calcium concentration, the patient had an episode of nephrolithiasis, which is a known complication related to the standard treatment of hypoparathyroidism with calcium and calcitriol. Calcium carbonate supplements were replaced by calcium citrate and hydrochlorothiazide was added to reduce urinary calcium excretion.

Currently, the patient still requires high doses of oral calcium and calcitriol to remain asymptomatic and to control her serum calcium concentration.

Patients with seizures precipitated by metabolic derangements may be at risk for seizure recurrence in the acute setting if the underlying metabolic disturbance is prolonged, thus, short-term antiseizure drug therapy can be considered [11]. However, several antiepileptic drugs, including carbamazepine, phenobarbital, and phenytoin, induce the cytochrome P450 system of liver enzymes, which increases the catabolism of 25-hydroxyvitamin D, and may have negative effects on serum calcium concentrations [13, 14]. Thus, these drugs should be used with caution in patients with hypoparathyroidism and hypocalcemia. Since the seizure was precipitated by hypocalcemia, the antiepileptic drug phenytoin was discontinued. While it remains a matter of clinical judgment, therapy with antiepileptic drugs may not be necessary for patients with epileptic seizures in the setting of hypocalcemia in hypoparathyroidism, even those with subcortical calcification [15, 16].

Outcome

Now 3 years postoperatively, she is on calcium citrate (4 g of elemental calcium in divided doses), 1.5 µg of calcitriol (in divided doses), 1,600 IU of cholecalciferol, 25 mg of hydrochlorothiazide, and 200 µg of levothyroxine daily. She has been compliant with her medications. The high cost of rhPTH(1–84) is a limitation for its use in this patient. Over the last 6 months, she has been asymptomatic, and her total calcium serum levels have ranged from 7.5 to 8.2 mg/dL. Her last urinary calcium was normal, serum phosphate was in the high-normal range, and serum PTH was still undetectable. She has had no further presentations with seizure.

Clinical Pearls and Pitfalls

- Seizures can occur in the setting of hypocalcemia, primarily generalized tonic-clonic and focal motor seizures.
- There is no correlation linking a specific serum calcium level to the seizure threshold or to EEG changes in hypocalcemia.
- Patients presenting with hypocalcemia and seizure should be treated acutely with intravenous calcium to raise serum calcium within the low-normal range.
- While it remains a matter of clinical judgment, treatment with antiepileptic drugs may not be needed for patients with epileptic seizures in the setting of hypocalcemia in hypoparathyroidism, even those with subcortical calcification.

Conflict of Interest   The authors declare no conflicts of interest.

References

1. Bilezikian JP, Brandi ML, Cusano NE, Mannstadt M, Rejnmark L, Rizzoli R, et al. Management of hypoparathyroidism: present and future. J Clin Endocrinol Metab. 2016;101(6):2313–24.
2. Armelisasso C, Vaccario ML, Pontecorvi A, Mazza S. Tonic-clonic seizures in a patient with primary hypoparathyroidism: a case report. Clin EEG Neurosci. 2004;35(2):97–9.
3. Kline CA, Esekogwu VI, Henderson SO, Newton KI. Non-convulsive status epilepticus in a patient with hypocalcemia. J Emerg Med. 1998;16(5):715–8.
4. Riggs JE. Neurologic manifestations of electrolyte disturbances. Neurol Clin. 2002;20(1):227–39, vii.
5. Seedat F, Daya R, Bhana SA. Hypoparathyroidism causing seizures: when epilepsy does not fit. Case Rep Med. 2018;2018:5948254.

6. Zuckermann EC, Glaser GH. Anticonvulsive action of increased calcium concentration in cerebrospinal fluid. Arch Neurol. 1973;29(4):245–52.

7. Swash M, Rowan AJ. Electroencephalographic criteria of hypocalcemia and hypercalcemia. Arch Neurol. 1972;26(3):218–28. PubMed PMID: 4536776.

8. Underbjerg L, Sikjaer T, Mosekilde L, Rejnmark L. Cardiovascular and renal complications to postsurgical hypoparathyroidism: a Danish nationwide controlled historic follow-up study. J Bone Miner Res. 2013;28(11):2277–85. PubMed PMID: 23661265.

9. Underbjerg L, Sikjaer T, Mosekilde L, Rejnmark L. The epidemiology of nonsurgical hypoparathyroidism in Denmark: a Nationwide Case Finding Study. J Bone Miner Res. 2015;30(9):1738–44. PubMed PMID: 25753591.

10. Vadiveloo T, Donnan PT, Leese CJ, Abraham KJ, Leese GP. Increased mortality and morbidity in patients with chronic hypoparathyroidism: a population-based study. Clin Endocrinol (Oxf). 2019;90:285–92.

11. Fields MC, Labovitz DL, French JA. Hospital-onset seizures: an inpatient study. JAMA Neurol. 2013;70(3):360–4.

12. Brandi ML, Bilezikian JP, Shoback D, Bouillon R, Clarke BL, Thakker RV, et al. Management of hypoparathyroidism: summary statement and guidelines. J Clin Endocrinol Metab. 2016;101(6):2273–83.

13. Menon B, Harinarayan CV. The effect of anti epileptic drug therapy on serum 25-hydroxyvitamin D and parameters of calcium and bone metabolism – a longitudinal study. Seizure. 2010;19(3):153–8.

14. Wang Z, Schuetz EG, Xu Y, Thummel KE. Interplay between vitamin D and the drug metabolizing enzyme CYP3A4. J Steroid Biochem Mol Biol. 2013;136:54–8. PubMed PMID: 22985909. Pubmed Central PMCID: 3549031.

15. Modi S, Tripathi M, Saha S, Goswami R. Seizures in patients with idiopathic hypoparathyroidism: effect of antiepileptic drug withdrawal on recurrence of seizures and serum calcium control. Eur J Endocrinol. 2014;170(5):777–83.

16. Liu MJ, Li JW, Shi XY, Hu LY, Zou LP. Epileptic seizure, as the first symptom of hypoparathyroidism in children, does not require antiepileptic drugs. Childs Nerv Syst. 2017;33(2):297–305.

Chapter 13
Hypoparathyroidism and Quality of Life

Tamara Vokes

Case Presentation

A 41-year-old woman was referred for possible participation in the clinical trial of rhPTH(1–84) for treatment of hypoparathyroidism known as REPLACE and described in detail in reference [1]. Seven years earlier, she had a thyroidectomy for papillary follicular carcinoma and developed hypoparathyroidism after surgery. Her thyroid cancer was treated with 150 mCi of I^{131}. Subsequent total body iodine scans were negative, and thyroglobulin was undetectable. For hypoparathyroidism she was taking 2250 mg of calcium and 1 mcg of calcitriol daily together with 4000 IU of native vitamin D. She complained of frequent twitching of the hands and face, tingling of the hands, fatigue, and inability to multitask. After enrolment in the clinical trial REPLACE, her rhPTH(1–84) doses were progressively increased from 50 to 75 and 100 mcg, while calcitriol was eliminated, and the dose of cal-

T. Vokes (✉)
Department of Medicine, Section of Endocrinology,
University of Chicago, Chicago, IL, USA
e-mail: tvokes@uchicago.edu

© Springer Nature Switzerland AG 2020
N. E. Cusano (ed.), *Hypoparathyroidism*,
https://doi.org/10.1007/978-3-030-29433-5_13

cium reduced to 750 mg per day at the end of the 6 month trial. The patient reported a remarkable improvement in her well-being with no further visits to the emergency room, improved energy, and ability to juggle multiple responsibilities resulting from working as a physical therapist and caring for her four children. She reported that while before starting rhPTH(1–84) she had to have "post-its everywhere" to be able to manage daily tasks, this was no longer the case when she was on the rhPTH(1–84) injections.

The SF-36 scores for this patient are shown in the following table.

Parameter	Baseline	End of study
Bodily pain	72	72
General health	57	62
Role-physical	100	100
Physical functioning	95	100
Physical component scores	50.9	51.3
Role-emotional	100	100
Mental health	80	95
Social functioning	100	100
Vitality	44	100
Mental component scores	52.1	62.3

Assessment and Diagnosis

In order to understand how to approach a patient who desires PTH therapy due to poor well-being, it is necessary to review what is known about quality of life (QOL) in hypoparathyroidism. This disease is often associated with multitude of complaints that indicate diminished QOL [2–4]. The complaints include impairments in multiple domains including physical (fatigue and low energy, pain and tightness, paresthesia, cramping, severe tetany and even seizures), emotional (depression, anxiety, personality disorders), and cognitive (poor memory and concentration, slow processing, inability to multitask, and poorly defined but popular among patients complaints of "brain fog"). It is not surprising that patients with hypoparathyroidism often do not feel well since normal serum calcium is necessary for many physiologic functions and is (in people with normal parathyroid function) maintained in a narrow range. In contrast, patients with hypoparathyroidism are asked to maintain blood calcium at or below the lower limit of normal, which is not a physiologic state. What is surprising, however, is the variability in the subjective experience of this disease. While there are patients who lead almost normal, productive lives (including running marathons), others are severely incapacitated, often unable to get out of bed in the morning, incapable of maintaining a gainful employment and satisfying social interactions. The reasons for these interindividual differences remain unclear and likely relate to underlying physical and mental health, difficulty in controlling serum calcium, and the quantity of oral supplements that the patient has to take to maintain serum calcium in the target range. The chronicity also seems to play a role as it is often observed that patients who have a slowly developing nonsurgical forms do not even come to medical attention for some time, while patients with hypoparathyroidism that develops after neck surgery often have severe symptoms.

Impairments in QOL in hypoparathyroidism have been recognized for a long time. Nevertheless, systematic studies of this problem are relatively recent and likely, at least in part, a result of the development of PTH and its analogs as potential replacement therapy. It should be noted that in all the studies cited below (with the exception of reference [5]), the control of serum calcium was at the level that would be considered adequate for this disease.

Several *case-control studies* reported lower quality of life in patients with hypoparathyroidism compared to either healthy controls or patients who are hypothyroid as a result of thyroid surgery but have retained normal parathyroid function. The earliest published study found that 25 women with both thyroid and parathyroid deficiency after surgery had higher global complaint scores compared to 25 women who only had hypothyroidism [6]. A similar, more recent study from Denmark compared 22 patients with surgical hypothyroidism and hypoparathyroidism, 22 patients with just surgical hypothyroidism, and 22 healthy matched controls [7]. The investigators found that hypoparathyroid patients had lower scores on the Short Form 36 Health Survey (SF-36), primarily in the physical domains, than the other two groups. A case-control study with an unusual design was conducted in the Harvard system [8]. SF-36 surveys were completed by 340 patients with surgical hypoparathyroidism, as well as 102 experienced endocrine surgeons and 200 healthy controls who were given a standard preoperative description of how hypoparathyroidism might feel. The patients with hypoparathyroidism scored significantly lower than the other two groups indicating that description of hypoparathyroidism as a possible complication of neck surgery (usually thyroid) given as a part of the surgical consenting process is inadequate. Furthermore, it became apparent that even experienced endocrine surgeons fail to appreciate the extent of suffering that might occur as a complication of surgery.

Several *epidemiologic studies* also uncovered lower QOL in hypoparathyroid patients compared to healthy controls. Examination of the Danish National Registry found that 688 patients with surgical hypoparathyroidism had more psychiatric symptoms than 1752 matched controls [9] and that 180 patients with nonsurgical hypoparathyroidism had a higher probability of neuropsychiatric disorders than 540 controls [10]. A Norwegian survey of 283 patients who responded (out of 522 who were invited) revealed that patients had worse scores on SF-36 as well as the Hospital Anxiety and Depression Scale and that patients with surgical forms were more impaired than those with the nonsurgical causes [11].

Finally, in all studies of QOL response to PTH therapy, baseline QOL scores were lower than in the general population [5, 12–16].

Management

Using PTH as hormone replacement in hypoparathyroidism held the promise of restoring both physiology and well-being. The results of the studies, however, have been inconsistent and although promising have fallen short of the expectations for restoration of normalcy. There are many reasons for this, not the least being the fact that the current modes of administration are far from physiologic replacement in that they do not result in sustained controlled levels of PTH in the circulation. However, they are certainly a very significant step forward, and many patients on PTH are tremendously appreciative of the improvement in the management of their disease, an anecdotal observation that is not completely consistent with the results of controlled studies.

Two groups have examined QOL response to PTH in studies with *open-label design* without a placebo comparator. A group from Columbia University in New York City administered SF-36 surveys to 54 patients before and 1, 2, 6, and 12 months after starting treatment with rhPTH(1–84) at 100 mcg every other day [13]. During the study, serum calcium was maintained in the target range, while the doses of supplements (calcium and calcitriol) were reduced by about half. QOL scores were low at baseline, improved after 1 month, and maintained for the duration of the study. This study was extended to 5 years with 69 enrolled patients [12]. However, the duration of follow-up varied: 5 years in 25, 4 years in 26, 3 years in 33, 2 years in 42, and 1 year in 58 patients. Overall, the study documented improved QOL over 5 years. However, it is important to appreciate that while some patients have not yet reached the 5-year mark, there were also 27 patients who dropped out for various reasons (not necessarily adverse events) and that these patients had lower QOL scores for at least some domains than those who remained in the study. This suggests at least some interindividual differences in the QOL response to PTH therapy.

The second open-label study was conducted in Italy where 42 subjects with surgical hypoparathyroidism were treated with PTH(1–34) at a dose of 20 mcg twice a day for 6 months [5]. In contrast to all other studies mentioned in this review, the control of calcium at baseline was suboptimal. As a result of study participation with adjustment of supplement doses and administration of PTH(1–34), mean serum calcium increased from an average of 7.6 to 8.9 mg/dL. Concurrently, SF-36 scores improved significantly in all domains, but the interpretation of the contribution of PTH(1–34) to well-being is less clear since it is possible that improving calcium levels by changing supplement doses would have resulted in a similar subjective benefit. This study was extended to 2 years during which the QOL was maintained although, at least for some domains, it was lower at 2 years than at 6 months [14].

There are also two studies that examined the QOL response to PTH in a *double-blind placebo-controlled design*. A study from Denmark examined QOL and muscle function in 32 patients who received 100 mcg of PTH(1–84) daily and 30 patients who injected a matching placebo for 6 months [15]. In this study, however, the doses of oral calcium and active vitamin D were reduced only if patients developed hypercalcemia which occurred in a significantly higher proportion of patients on PTH. Neither QOL nor objective tests of muscle function showed a significant benefit from PTH therapy, possibly because hypercalcemia may have had a negative effect on these outcomes.

The second double-blind placebo-controlled study was REPLACE, a multicenter, international registration trial that led to the approval of rhPTH(1–84) for treatment of adult patients with hypoparathyroidism in the USA [16]. In contrast to the Danish trial with a fixed PTH dose, in REPLACE the approach was to maintain serum calcium in the target range through progressive increase in the rhPTH(1–84) dose (from 50 to 75 and a maximum of 100 mcg/day) and reduction in the supplement doses. Because this was effectively accomplished in the trial, serum calcium was similar in the placebo- and PTH-treated groups both at the beginning and at the end of the 6-month trial. In response to treatment, SF-36 scores improved in several domains in the PTH-treated but not in placebo-treated patients. However, the difference between the groups was not statistically significant. Interestingly, there was a significant interaction between the response and the geographic region with North America and Western Europe showing a greater improvement with PTH therapy and significant differences between PTH- and placebo-treated patients, while patients from Hungary did not have any improvement in the SF-36 scores. It is not clear whether this discrepancy may have been due to misunderstanding of the Hungarian translation by the patients.

The logical question arising from the above studies is whether we have firm evidence of the effectiveness of PTH in improving QOL that would justify the cost of such treatment [17]. While the results of the studies are inconsistent, it is clear that at least some patients experience a dramatic improvement in well-being with this therapy (as illustrated by the case presentation above). The predictors of improvement are not entirely clear. REPLACE investigators did look for such predictors and found that patients with greater impairment in QOL at baseline (lower SF-36 scores) had greater improvement in response to PTH [16]. There was also some association, although considerably less strong than baseline QOL, between the changes in SF-36 scores and the reduction in supplement doses with patients with greater decrease in the daily number of pills scoring higher on SF-36 testing. Based on these observations, it appears that patients who have poor QOL on conventional therapy and/or require large doses of supplements would most benefit from addition of PTH therapy. The case above also illustrates that the objective assessment of QOL is challenging and likely will require a development of disease-specific instruments. In addition, further investigation into the mechanism of QOL impairments and their correlation with biochemical alterations, if any, is warranted.

Outcome

This patient reported (transcribed from a videotaped interview by a medical student): "Functioning without parathyroids is incredible. It starts gradually, you get tingles and difficulty feeling your feet, then you lose strength in your legs and arms and you can't stand up and you can't move, you can't talk and at that point if you do not get calcium in you quickly then you can't move at all and your heart can stop. It has happened to me 6 times before I was on PTH. Since I got the dose right I get tingles now and then but nothing like before."

As we can see from the above example, despite the mostly negligible increase in the SF-36 scores (except for vitality which did improve), the patient reports her well-being as markedly improved.

Clinical Pearls and Pitfalls
- Quality of life is often impaired in hypoparathyroidism with signficant inter-individual differences in the degree of impairment.
- Addition of PTH therapy to conventional treatment with calcium and active vitamin D has shown improvement in quality of life at least in some studies.
- Greater improvements with PTH therapy seem to occur in patients who have the lowest quality of life indices on conventional therapy.

Conflict of Interest   The authors declare no conflicts of interest.

References

1. Mannstadt M, et al. Efficacy and safety of recombinant human parathyroid hormone (1-84) in hypoparathyroidism (REPLACE): a double-blind, placebo-controlled, randomised, phase 3 study. Lancet Diabetes Endocrinol. 2013;1(4):275–83.
2. Buttner M, Musholt TJ, Singer S. Quality of life in patients with hypoparathyroidism receiving standard treatment: a systematic review. Endocrine. 2017;58(1):14–20.

3. Shoback D. Clinical practice. Hypoparathyroidism. N Engl J Med. 2008;359(4):391–403.
4. Shoback DM, et al. Presentation of hypoparathyroidism: etiologies and clinical features. J Clin Endocrinol Metab. 2016;101(6):2300–12.
5. Santonati A, et al. PTH(1-34) for surgical hypoparathyroidism: a prospective, open-label investigation of efficacy and quality of life. J Clin Endocrinol Metab. 2015;100(9):3590–7.
6. Arlt W, et al. Well-being, mood and calcium homeostasis in patients with hypoparathyroidism receiving standard treatment with calcium and vitamin D. Eur J Endocrinol. 2002;146(2):215–22.
7. Sikjaer T, et al. Concurrent hypoparathyroidism is associated with impaired physical function and quality of life in hypothyroidism. J Bone Miner Res. 2016;31(7):1440–8.
8. Cho NL, et al. Surgeons and patients disagree on the potential consequences from hypoparathyroidism. Endocr Pract. 2014;20(5):427–46.
9. Underbjerg L, et al. Postsurgical hypoparathyroidism – risk of fractures, psychiatric diseases, cancer, cataract, and infections. J Bone Miner Res. 2014;29(11):2504–10.
10. Underbjerg L, et al. The epidemiology of nonsurgical hypoparathyroidism in Denmark: a Nationwide Case Finding Study. J Bone Miner Res. 2015;30(9):1738–44.
11. Astor MC, et al. Epidemiology and health-related quality of life in hypoparathyroidism in Norway. J Clin Endocrinol Metab. 2016;101(8):3045–53.
12. Cusano NE, et al. PTH(1-84) is associated with improved quality of life in hypoparathyroidism through 5 years of therapy. J Clin Endocrinol Metab. 2014;99(10):3694–9.
13. Cusano NE, et al. The effect of PTH(1-84) on quality of life in hypoparathyroidism. J Clin Endocrinol Metab. 2013;98(6):2356–61.
14. Palermo A, et al. PTH(1-34) for surgical hypoparathyroidism: a 2-year prospective, open-label investigation of efficacy and quality of life. J Clin Endocrinol Metab. 2018;103(1):271–80.
15. Sikjaer T, et al. Effects of PTH(1-84) therapy on muscle function and quality of life in hypoparathyroidism: results from a randomized controlled trial. Osteoporos Int. 2014;25(6):1717–26.
16. Vokes TJ, et al. Recombinant human parathyroid hormone effect on health-related quality of life in adults with chronic hypoparathyroidism. J Clin Endocrinol Metab. 2018;103(2):722–31.
17. Winer KK. Does PTH replacement therapy improve quality of life in patients with chronic hypoparathyroidism? J Clin Endocrinol Metab. 2018;103(7):2752–5.

Chapter 14
Hypoparathyroidism and the Skeleton

Tanja Sikjaer

Case Presentation

A 54-year-old woman had a total thyroidectomy. She had an enlarged atoxic goiter since the age of 19, and due to continous growth of the goiter, she had it removed for cosmetic reasons in 1995. After surgery, she developed tetany due to hypocalcemia and was diagnosed with postsurgical hypoparathyroidism. Initially only calcium supplements were initiated, but very shortly after she also started treatment with activated vitamin D (alfacalcidol). During follow-up she had measurable but low levels of PTH in combination with hypocalcemia. She had no other diseases affecting the skeleton or calcium homeostasis.

Due to inclusion in a clinical trial, she had an extensive diagnostic evaluation performed in 2009 at the age of 67. At the time of investigation, she had been diagnosed with hypoparathyroidism for 14 years and was treated with 0.5 µg alfacalcidol and 2000 mg of calcium supplements daily.

T. Sikjaer (✉)
Department of Endocrinology and Internal Medicine,
Aarhus University Hospital, Aarhus, Denmark
e-mail: Tansik@rm.dk

© Springer Nature Switzerland AG 2020
N. E. Cusano (ed.), *Hypoparathyroidism*,
https://doi.org/10.1007/978-3-030-29433-5_14

Bone mineral density (BMD) was measured both as areal BMD (g/cm^2) by dual-energy X-ray absorptiometry (DXA) and as volumetric BMD (vBMD, mg/cm^3) by quantitative computed tomography (QCT).

By DXA, she had a T-score of +3.9 at the spine L1-L2 (L3 + L4 excluded due to arthritis), +1.2 at the total hip and +0.6 at the forearm. By QCT, she had a calculated T-score of +1.3 at the spine (L1-L2) and +0.8 at the total hip. Both scans show that the patient had very dense bone at the age of 67.

Furthermore, the patient had plasma and urine bone turnover markers measured, showing low or low-normal values. Formation markers were relatively suppressed osteocalcin = 8 ug/L (reference: 13–55 ug/L), propeptide of type 1 collagen (P1NP) = 6 µg/L (reference: <93 µg/L) and bone-specific alkaline phosphatase (BAP) = 19 U/L (reference: 12–50 U/L). Bone resorption markers were also low normal, including C-telopeptide CTx = 0.05 µg/L (reference 0.03–0.83 µg/L) and urine N-telopeptide (U-NTx/Cr) = 17 × 10^{-6} (reference: 17–94 × 10^{-6} nmol BCE/mmol creatinine).

Concerning fractures, the patient has only had a tarsal fracture in the right foot at 30 years of age and none after acquiring hypoparathyroidism.

In 2009, she started treatment with subcutaneous injections of rhPTH(1–84) 100 µg once a day.

Assessment and Diagnosis

PTH is a key regulator in bone remodelling, and when it is either missing or at insufficient levels, it has a marked effect on the skeleton. Using histomorphometry, Langdahl et al. [1] showed reduced bone turnover in 12 patients with hypoparathyroidism compared to 13 age- and gender-matched normal controls. The study showed a reduced resorption rate with a prolonged resorption period and a reduced resorption depth. Moreover, they found a prolonged quiescent period and a reduced activation frequency. These observations have been confirmed by Rubin et al. [2] in 33 patients with hypoparathyroidism. Results from both studies are very much in line with the findings of bone turnover markers abnormally low or low within the reference range in several studies of hypoparathyroidism [3–6]. The low activity of bone remodelling, both formation and resorption, may over time lead to an increased BMD in these patients. Several studies have demonstrated high T- and Z-scores with the highest scores in the lumbar spine [2, 3, 5, 7–10]. Looking at bone microarchitecture by high-resolution peripheral quantitative computed tomography (HRpQCT), micro-computed tomography (μ-CT) and histomorphometry, several studies have been performed. Cusano et al. [9] performed HRpQCT on 60 men and women with hypoparathyroidism and found a higher cortical vBMD at both the tibia and radius including a reduced cortical porosity (pre- and postmenopausal women) compared to a normative control group. At the trabecular site, they found results that were more mixed. Trabecular numbers at the tibia were higher in the hypoparathyroid young women (<40 years) and young men (<50 years). In the young women, there were also lower trabecular thickness and separation. In a study by Underbjerg et al. [5], 58 patients with non-surgical hypoparathyroidism were compared to age- and gender-matched healthy controls, and the patients were found to have a higher total and cortical area as well as cortical vBMD and thickness at both the radius and tibia. There were no difference in cortical porosity or any trabecular indices. Using HRpQCT it seems that the abnormal bone architecture is mainly at the cortical site. Using μ-CT, Rubin et al. [11] compared bone biopsies from 25 patients with hypoparathyroidism with 25 controls (13 living and 12 cadavers) without bone disease. They found a greater trabecular thickness, trabecular number and connectivity density in the patients with hypoparathyroidism. When they added more patients (total $n = 33$) and more controls (total cadavers $n = 36$), the biopsies were no longer matched on age and gender, but they found a greater cancellous bone volume, while trabecular separation and structural modelling index (SMI) were significantly lower. These findings are in agreement with the findings by histomorphometry in the same 33 patients with hypoparathyroidism as mentioned above.

As shown above only a few studies have compared bone architecture in hypoparathyroid patients to controls without bone disease. The findings by HRpQCT, μ-CT and histomorphometry describe abnormalities at both cortical and trabecular sites.

It has been speculated whether reduced bone remodelling in hypoparathyroidism could lead to old, dense bones with lower strength due to less repair of microcracks and skeletal abnormalities. There have only been a few studies on fracture risk in patients with hypoparathyroidism. Underbjerg et al. have performed two historic cohort studies [12, 13], based on hospital discharge codes. In the first study, 688 patients with post-surgical hyperparathyroidism were included and compared to 2063 age- and gender-matched controls. In the second study, 180 patients with non-surgical hypopathyroidism were identified and compared with 540 age- and gender-matched controls. There were no overall differences in fracture risk between the groups, but looking at fracture types, there was a reduced fracture risk at the proximal humerus (HR 0.69, 95% CI 0.49–0.97) in the postsurgical hypoparathyroid patients, whereas there was an increased risk at the humerus (HR 1.93; 95% CI, 1.31; 2.85) in the non-surgical hypoparathyroid patients. In a study by Mitchell et al. [10], they identified 120 patients with hypoparathyroidism diagnosed for at least 1 year. Twenty-one (18%) of the patients sustained a fracture during 7 years of follow-up. The fractures occurred at ten different skeletal sites, and two traumatic incidents were included (fall from stairs and motor vehicle rollover). The study did not compare fracture risk to a control group or the background population. The studies of HRpQCT in hypoparathyroidism [5, 9, 14] showed no difference in simulated stress by calculated finite element analyses between patients with hypoparathyroidism and controls.

Management

PTH therapy in hypoparathyroidism has been shown to increase the reduced bone turnover in the disease. Several studies [3, 15–17] have shown a marked increase in both bone formation and resorption markers. The rise depends on the compound [PTH(1–34) or rhPTH(1–84)], the daily dose and the method of administration (subcutaneous injection or by pump therapy). With the highest dose of 100 μg rhPTH(1–84) once a day, Sikjaer et al. [3] showed an increase in BAP (226% ± 36%), osteocalcin (+807% ± 186%), P1NP (1315% ± 330%), CTx (1209% ± 459%) and U-NTx/Cr (830% ± 165%). When administered continuously by pump, [18], bone markers only normalized and did not reach levels above the reference range. Long-term data exist from two studies, the first a three-year study of PTH(1–34) by Winer et al. [16] where they found continuously increased levels of both formation and resorption markers above the reference range but with a downward trend of the curve after 2.5 years of treatment. The second study by Rubin et al. [19] was performed using rhPTH(1–84) initially with 100 μg every second day and they showed an up to three-fold increase in bone markers after 1 year with a decrease over time ending up after 6 years of treatment with levels that remained above baselines values, but within the reference range.

Concerning BMD changes with PTH treatment, it probably also depends on the compound, dosing and length of treatment. In the study by Sikjaer et al. [3], BMD decreased at the hip, spine and whole body after 6 months of treatment. Nine patients continued rhPTH(1–84) for another 2 years and regained the loss of BMD resulting in no difference at the spine, total hip or whole body but a decrease at the forearm after a total of 2.5 years of treatment compared to the control group on conventional treatment [20]. Three years of treatment with PTH(1–34) did not show any significant between-group differences but a non-significant downward trend in the PTH-treated group ($P = 0.06$) at the distal one-third radius [16]. The longest data existing on BMD changes is the 6-year data from Rubin et al. [19] showing an increase at the spine ($3.8 \pm 1\%$, $P = 0.004$) and the total hip ($2.4 \pm 1\%$, $P = 0.02$) but a decrease at the distal one-third radius ($-4.4 \pm 1\%$, $P < 0.0001$).

There are no solid data on whether PTH treatment changes the risk of fractures. After 6 years of treatment, Rubin et al. [19] had recorded eight fractures in six patients (total N = 33) but with an even distribution over time, with the first fracture during the first year of treatment.

In the case of postsurgical hypoparathyroidism, a DXA scan can be performed as a diagnostic work-up at the time of diagnosis. In the case of osteopenia or normal values, there is no need for routine monitoring of the bone due to hypoparathyroidism being a state of very low bone turnover, and BMD is not expected to decrease during the course of the disease. In the case of other disorders or drug therapies (e.g. glucocorticoids), guidelines for when to repeat measurements should follow the recommendations of the International Society of Clinical Densitometry [21]. Antiresorptive treatments are rarely needed, as hypoparathyroidism is a state of (very) low bone turnover.

Outcome

After 6 months of treatment with rhPTH(1–84), the abnormally low bone remodelling was increased as measured by bone markers. Her formation markers increased markedly. Osteocalcin increased by 452%, PINP by 1749% and BAP by 227%. Bone resorption also increased demonstrated by an increase in CTx of 1416% and U-NTx/Cr of 69%. Bone markers were measured again after a total of 2.5 years of treatment with rhPTH(1–84). Osteocalcin and PINP were still above the reference range with values of 170 μg/L and 272 μg/L, respectively. BAP had decreased again and was within the reference range. CTx and U-NTx/Cr were also continuously elevated with 1.32 μg/l and 227 ×10^{-6} nmol BCE/mmol Cr, respectively.

DXA after 2.5 years of treatment showed insignificant changes in BMD with +0.6% at the spine (L1-L2), −2.7% at the total hip and −2.1% at the total forearm.

After 3 years of rhPTH(1–84) treatment, her dose was reduced to 100 μg every second day, and she continued this treatment for an additional 4 months until the product was taken off the market.

No fractures occurred after a total of 3 years and 4 months of treatment with rhPTH(1–84).

Clinical Pearls and Pitfalls
- Due to very low bone turnover, bone mass is often high in patients with hypoparathyroidism, and osteoporosis in these patients is rare. In the case of osteoporosis, the effect of antiresorptive treatment is probably minimal due to the already low bone turnover.
- There is no need for following patients with regular DXA scans because of low bone turnover.
- There is no evidence for a difference in fracture risk in patients with hypoparathyroidism compared to the background population.
- When initiating PTH treatment, there will be an expected increase in bone turnover markers, and there might be an initial decrease in BMD, which will increase again in the long term at the hip and spine.

Conflict of Interest   The authors declare no conflicts of interest.

References

1. Langdahl BL, Mortensen L, Vesterby A, Eriksen EF, Charles P. Bone histomorphometry in hypoparathyroid patients treated with vitamin D. Bone. 1996;18(2):103–8.
2. Rubin MR, Dempster DW, Zhou H, Shane E, Nickolas T, Sliney J Jr, et al. Dynamic and structural properties of the skeleton in hypoparathyroidism. J Bone Miner Res. 2008;23(12):2018–24.
3. Sikjaer T, Rejnmark L, Rolighed L, Heickendorff L, Mosekilde L. The effect of adding PTH(1-84) to conventional treatment of hypoparathyroidism: a randomized, placebo-controlled study. J Bone Miner Res. 2011;26(10):2358–70.
4. Kruse K, Kracht U, Wohlfart K, Kruse U. Biochemical markers of bone turnover, intact serum parathyroid horn and renal calcium excretion in patients with pseudohypoparathyroidism

and hypoparathyroidism before and during vitamin D treatment. Eur J Pediatr. 1989;148(6):535–9.

5. Underbjerg L, Malmstroem S, Sikjaer T, Rejnmark L. Bone status among patients with nonsurgical hypoparathyroidism, autosomal dominant hypocalcaemia, and pseudohypoparathyroidism: a cohort study. J Bone Miner Res. 2018;33:467.

6. Rubin MR, Dempster DW, Sliney J Jr, Zhou H, Nickolas TL, Stein EM, et al. PTH(1-84) administration reverses abnormal bone-remodeling dynamics and structure in hypoparathyroidism. J Bone Miner Res. 2011;26(11):2727–36.

7. Abugassa S. Bone mineral density in patients with chronic hypoparathyroidism. J Clin Endocrinol Metab. 1993;76(6):1617–21.

8. Seeman E, Wahner HW, Offord KP, Kumar R, Johnson WJ, Riggs BL. Differential effects of endocrine dysfunction on the axial and the appendicular skeleton. J Clin Invest. 1982;69(6):1302–9.

9. Cusano NE, Nishiyama KK, Zhang C, Rubin MR, Boutroy S, McMahon DJ, et al. Noninvasive assessment of skeletal microstructure and estimated bone strength in hypoparathyroidism. J Bone Miner Res. 2016;31(2):308–16.

10. Mitchell DM, Regan S, Cooley MR, Lauter KB, Vrla MC, Becker CB, et al. Long-term follow-up of patients with hypoparathyroidism. J Clin Endocrinol Metab. 2012;97(12):4507–14. Epub 2012/10/09.

11. Rubin MR, Dempster DW, Kohler T, Stauber M, Zhou H, Shane E, et al. Three dimensional cancellous bone structure in hypoparathyroidism. Bone. 2010;46(1):190–5.

12. Underbjerg L, Sikjaer T, Mosekilde L, Rejnmark L. Postsurgical hypoparathyroidism – risk of fractures, psychiatric diseases, cancer, cataract, and infections. J Bone Miner Res. 2014;29(11):2504–10.

13. Underbjerg L, Sikjaer T, Mosekilde L, Rejnmark L. The epidemiology of nonsurgical hypoparathyroidism in Denmark: a Nationwide case finding study. J Bone Miner Res. 2015;30(9):1738–44.

14. Cohen A, Dempster DW, Muller R, Guo XE, Nickolas TL, Liu XS, et al. Assessment of trabecular and cortical architecture and mechanical competence of bone by high-resolution peripheral computed tomography: comparison with transiliac bone biopsy. Osteoporos Int. 2010;21(2):263–73.

15. Cusano NE, Rubin MR, McMahon DJ, Zhang C, Ives R, Tulley A, et al. Therapy of hypoparathyroidism with PTH(1-84): a

prospective four-year investigation of efficacy and safety. J Clin Endocrinol Metab. 2013;98(1):137–44.
16. Winer KK, Ko CW, Reynolds JC, Dowdy K, Keil M, Peterson D, et al. Long-term treatment of hypoparathyroidism: a randomized controlled study comparing parathyroid hormone-(1-34) versus calcitriol and calcium. J Clin Endocrinol Metab. 2003;88(9):4214–20.
17. Gafni RI, Brahim JS, Andreopoulou P, Bhattacharyya N, Kelly MH, Brillante BA, et al. Daily parathyroid hormone 1-34 replacement therapy for hypoparathyroidism induces marked changes in bone turnover and structure. J Bone Miner Res. 2012;27:1811.
18. Winer KK, Fulton KA, Albert PS, Cutler GB Jr. Effects of pump versus twice-daily injection delivery of synthetic parathyroid hormone 1-34 in children with severe congenital hypoparathyroidism. J Pediatr. 2014;165(3):556–63.e1. Epub 2014/06/21.
19. Rubin MR, Cusano NE, Fan WW, Delgado Y, Zhang C, Costa AG, et al. Therapy of hypoparathyroidism with PTH(1-84): a prospective six year investigation of efficacy and safety. J Clin Endocrinol Metab. 2016;101(7):2742–50. Epub 2016/05/05.
20. Sikjaer T, Moser E, L M. Effects of long term PTH(1-84) replacement therapy in hypoparathyroidism and the consequence of termination of therapy (Abstract SA0176). 2013 annual meeting of the American Society for Bone and Mineral Research. Baltimore, MD October 4–7, 2013: Journal of Bone and Mineral reseach; 2013. p. S1–S.
21. Schousboe JT, Shepherd JA, Bilezikian JP, Baim S. Executive summary of the 2013 International Society for Clinical Densitometry Position Development Conference on bone densitometry. J Clin Densitom. 2013;16(4):455–66. Epub 2013/11/05.

Chapter 15
Hypoparathyroidism in Pregnancy

Yousef Alalawi, Iman M'Hiri, Hajar Abu Alrob, and Aliya Khan

Case Presentation

A 36-year-old 8 weeks pregnant woman is referred for assessment of postsurgical hypoparathyroidism. She had a thyroidectomy completed 6 years ago and has been referred for management of hypoparathyroidism during pregnancy. She has a history of a prior miscarriage last year at 30 weeks gestation and is concerned that she may miscarry again. She had passed a renal stone at 20 weeks gestation at that time. She is otherwise well.

Currently, she has numbness and tingling in the face and hands occurring 2–3 times a week and also has muscle cramps in her legs a few times a month.

Y. Alalawi · H. A. Alrob · A. Khan (✉)
McMaster University, Hamilton, ON, Canada
e-mail: Aliya@mcmaster.ca

I. M'Hiri
Bone Research and Education Centre, Oakville, ON, Canada

© Springer Nature Switzerland AG 2020   143
N. E. Cusano (ed.), *Hypoparathyroidism*,
https://doi.org/10.1007/978-3-030-29433-5_15

No prior seizures or cardiac or respiratory complications from hypocalcemia.

Her medications included calcitriol 0.5 ug twice daily, calcium carbonate 1000 mg three times daily with meals, vitamin D 1000 IU daily, and levothyroxine 100 ug daily.

Her examination was significant for blood pressure 100/60 mmHg, pulse 60 beats per minute, Chvostek's sign negative, remainder of examination noncontributory. Her laboratory values are as per the table below.

Laboratory value	SI units	Imperial units
Ionized calcium	1 mmol/L low	4.00 mg/dL low
PTH	<0.6 pmol/L low	<5.68 pg/mL low
25-hydroxyvitamin D	90 nmol/L	36.1 ng/mL
eGFR	111 mL/min	111 mL/min/1.73 m^2
Magnesium	0.75 mmol/L	1.8 mg/dL
Phosphate	1.67 mmol/L high	5.17 mg/dL high
Urine calcium	10.3 mmol/day high	412.8 mg/24 hr high

Assessment and Diagnosis

Hypoparathyroidism is characterized by absent or inadequate parathyroid hormone (PTH) levels resulting in hypocalcemia and often hyperphosphatemia [1, 2]. Hypoparathyroidism during pregnancy may be associated with significant maternal and fetal morbidity as well as fetal losses, and close monitoring of serum calcium is required during pregnancy [3, 4]. Frequent adjustments in the doses of calcium and calcitriol may be necessary to avoid hypocalcemia as well as hypercalcemia and to optimize maternal and fetal outcomes [1].

Physiologic changes occur during pregnancy which affect serum calcium as well as the calcium-regulating hormones. These changes impact the care of our patients with hypoparathyroidism during pregnancy and must be taken into consideration when evaluating the results of the laboratory profile and in adjusting the doses of calcium supplements as well as additional drug therapy.

During pregnancy the intravascular volume increases and is associated with a decrease in serum albumin as well as a decrease in total albumin bound calcium. The ionized calcium, however, remains normal, and the calcium corrected for albumin is also normal [5–7]. Thus, it is essential to correct the serum calcium for the serum albumin prior to making any changes in management as the uncorrected serum calcium will appear to be falsely low. Serum phosphorus is unchanged during pregnancy [5–7]. In the first trimester, PTH is suppressed and falls into the low-normal reference range or even below the normal reference range in the first trimester [5–9]. PTH subsequently rises into the mid-normal reference range in the third trimester [10]. Maternal calcium intake from dietary sources as well as vitamin D levels will impact serum PTH.

Calcitriol levels increase in the first trimester by approximately two to threefold and may result in improved symptoms of hypocalcemia in women with hypoparathyroidism [6, 7, 10–12]. The rises in calcitriol enhance intestinal calcium absorption and suppress PTH [10]. Calcitriol is produced by the maternal kidneys as well as the placenta. During pregnancy, there is upregulation in the renal expression of Cyp27b1 which results in increased production of 1,25-dihydroxyvitamin D [1]. Elevations in serum calcitriol enhance increased intestinal calcium absorption and subsequently increase renal calcium filtration and increase urine calcium excretion [13]. Serum calcitonin also appears to increase during pregnancy and may protect the maternal skeleton from demineralization [5, 7, 10].

Longitudinal studies have shown rises in PTH related peptide (PTHrP) by approximately three times the baseline prepregnancy levels, and these rises begin in the first trimester [14]. Elevations in PTHrP may suppress PTH and upregulate calcitriol. The source for the elevations in PTHrP appears to be the placenta [10, 15]. Figure 15.1 presents a schematic overview of the changes in the calcium-regulating hormones during a normal pregnancy [16].

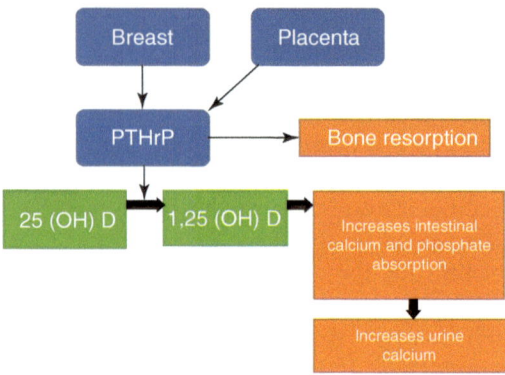

FIGURE 15.1 Calcium Homeostasis During Pregnancy-reproduced with permission from Khan et al. [1])

Hypercalciuria is often present in individuals with hypoparathyroidism due to the lack of PTH. The currently limited data suggest that urine calcium rises further during pregnancy in hypoparathyroid mothers in association with elevations in calcitriol, and this may increase the risk of renal stones during pregnancy particularly in the presence of low PTH [13, 17].

Our patient has postsurgical hypoparathyroidism – this diagnosis is confirmed by the presence of hypocalcemia in the presence of a low or absent PTH. It is important to evaluate serum magnesium as hypermagnesemia can bind to the calcium-sensing receptor and lower serum PTH. Low magnesium can impair PTH secretion and result in a tissue resistance to the effects of PTH and can contribute to low serum calcium [2]. Her magnesium is normal. She has hypercalciuria which is a reflection of the low PTH and she is at an increased risk of renal stones. Her history indicates that she had renal stones during her previous pregnancy. The serum phosphate is elevated and is consistent with a diagnosis of hypoparathyroidism.

Our evaluation will include a review of symptoms of hypocalcemia which include numbness, tingling of the face, hands, and feet as well as muscle cramps. It will be important to quantify how often these symptoms are experienced. Significant hypocalcemia can be associated with confusion, tetany, seizures, laryngospasm, bronchospasm, and carpal spasm. Cardiac arrhythmias may also occur with hypocalcemia, and rarely congestive heart failure can develop with significant reductions in serum calcium [18, 19]. In pregnancy, hypocalcemia is associated with uterine contractions, and if uterine contractions are present, it is important to closely monitor the serum calcium and administer higher doses of calcium supplements and possibly also a higher dose of calcitriol, recognizing that the laboratory test results reflect only the values at that point in time and serum calcium may fluctuate and may be lower at other time periods [1, 2].

The physical exam will include an evaluation of clinical features of hypocalcemia which include assessing the Chvostek's sign (tap cheek 2 cm anterior to the ear lobe and observe for ipsilateral twitching of the upper lip) and Trousseau's sign (elevate the blood pressure cuff above systolic for 3 min, and observe for carpal spasm).

Management

Due to the physiologic changes in the calcium-regulating hormones, some women may require lower doses of calcitriol and calcium supplementation, whereas other women may require higher doses as the skeletal needs of the fetus must be met. The variation in requirements of calcium and calcitriol may be due to multiple factors including variations in maternal renal expression of calcitonin, differences in dietary calcium intake, as well as variability in PTHrP secretion by the placenta and breasts during pregnancy in women with hypoparathyroidism [1].

It is difficult to predict who will require higher or lower doses of calcium and calcitriol supplementation. Therefore, it is recommended that all patients be closely followed with monitoring of serum calcium, phosphate, and serum magnesium during pregnancy. Inadequate calcium and calcitriol intake can contribute to inadequate mineral accrual in the developing fetal skeleton. Calcium, magnesium, and phosphorus are all actively transported by the placenta from the mother to the fetus against their concentration gradient to ensure optimal fetal skeletal health and calcification [20]. The fetal skeleton mineralizes over the course of gestation; however, mineral accrual predominantly occurs during the third trimester at which time approximately 80% of mineral accrual takes place [21]. The placenta delivers the essential nutrients – calcium, phosphate, and magnesium from maternal circulation to the fetus enabling fetal bone mineralization. Hypocalcemia in the mother will stimulate the fetal parathyroid glands and result in the development of hyperparathyroidism in the fetus with demineralization of the fetal skeleton [22–27]. Severe cases of fetal hyperparathyroidism present with bowing of the long bones, subperiosteal bone resorption, intrauterine rib and limb fractures, osteitis fibrosa cystica, spontaneous abortion, and low birth weight and can also result in fetal death [26]. Overtreatment of hypoparathyroidism with hypercalcemia in the mother will, however, result in increased calcium transport to the fetus with suppression of fetal parathyroid glands [27].

Hypocalcemia and hypercalcemia must be avoided to ensure the development of normal parathyroid function in the fetus. Uncorrected hypocalcemia has been shown to increase the risk of abortion [2]. Hypercalcemia must be avoided to prevent suppression of the fetal parathyroid glands. Intrauterine hypoparathyroidism has been associated with neonatal tetany [28]. Evidence-based recommendations advise monitoring serum calcium every 3–4 weeks during pregnancy to ensure that the serum calcium is maintained in the low-normal reference range [1, 2]. If changes in the doses of calcium or calcitriol are required, then the laboratory profile should be repeated in 1–2 weeks. As the half-life of calcitriol is 4–6 hours, steady state is achieved in five half-lives, and close monitoring will ensure that the serum calcium is maintained in the low-normal reference range. Calcitriol, vitamin D, and calcium are all approved and safe to use during pregnancy. PTH and thiazide diuretics should be discontinued. There is inadequate safety data regarding the use of PTH in pregnancy. The FDA classifies PTH as a category C drug. Thiazide diuretics are classified as a category B drug by the FDA [29].

Serum calcium should be measured postpartum within the first week and then weekly for the first month after childbirth. If mothers choose to breastfeed, then serum measures can be monitored monthly. If the fetus was exposed to prolonged periods of hypocalcemia or hypercalcemia, then the baby should be carefully monitored immediately following birth due to the increased risk of hypocalcemia or hypercalcemia [18, 30, 31].

Outcome

Our patient had her serum calcium followed every 2–3 weeks during pregnancy. Her uterine contractions resolved with increased calcium supplementation and a further increase in the dose of calcitriol to 0.75 ug in the morning and 0.5 ug in the afternoon. Serum calcium rose to the mid-normal reference range, and she remained asymptomatic during the rest of her pregnancy. At 38 weeks gestation, she went into labor and delivered a healthy male infant with normal Apgar scores and a normal serum calcium.

Clinical Pearls and Pitfalls

- Hypoparathyroidism during pregnancy is associated with significant morbidity for both the mother and the baby, as well as it is associated with an increased risk of abortion.
- Pregnant women with hypoparathyroidism require close monitoring of serum calcium aiming for a low-normal to mid-normal serum calcium.

- It is important to ensure that symptoms of hypocalcemia are treated, and the doses of calcium and calcitriol are appropriately increased in the presence of premature uterine contractions aiming for a serum calcium in the low-normal to mid-normal reference range.
- Avoidance of hypocalcemia as well as hypercalcemia is essential for the development of normal parathyroid function in the fetus.
- A multidisciplinary team approach with close coordination of care by the primary care physician, endocrinologist, pediatrician, and obstetrician is essential for the optimization of the maternal and neonatal outcomes.

Conflict of Interest   The authors declare no conflicts of interest.

References

1. Khan AA, Clarke B, Rejnmark L, Brandi ML. Management of endocrine disease: hypoparathyroidism in pregnancy: review and evidence-based recommendations for management. Eur J Endocrinol. 2019;180:R37. https://doi.org/10.1530/eje-18-0541.
2. Khan AA, Koch CA, Uum SV, Baillargeon JP, Bollerslev J, Brandi ML, et al. Standards of care for hypoparathyroidism in adults: a Canadian and International Consensus. Eur J Endocrinol. 2019;180:1–23. https://doi.org/10.1530/eje-18-0609.
3. Callies F, Arlt W, Scholz H, Reincke M, Allolio B. Management of hypoparathyroidism during pregnancy: report of twelve cases. Eur J Endocrinol. 1998;139(3):284–9. https://doi.org/10.1530/eje.0.1390284.
4. Eastell R, Edmonds CJ, Chayal RC, Mcfadyen IR. Prolonged hypoparathyroidism presenting eventually as second trimester abortion. Br Med J. 1985;291(6500):955–6. https://doi.org/10.1136/bmj.291.6500.955.

5. Dahlman T, Sjöberg HE, Bucht E. Calcium homeostasis in normal pregnancy and puerperium: a longitudinal study. Acta Obstet Gynecol Scand. 1994;73(5):393–8. https://doi.org/10.3109/00016349409006250.

6. Seki K, Makimura N, Mitsui C, Hirata J, Nagata I. Calcium-regulating hormones and osteocalcin levels during pregnancy: a longitudinal study. Am J Obstet Gynecol. 1991;164(5):1248–52. https://doi.org/10.1016/0002-9378(91)90694-m.

7. Ardawi M, Nasrat H, Baaqueel H. Calcium-regulating hormones and parathyroid hormone-related peptide in normal human pregnancy and postpartum: a longitudinal study. Eur J Endocrinol. 1997;137:402–9. https://doi.org/10.1530/eje.0.1370402.

8. Black AJ, Topping J, Durham B, Farquharson RG, Fraser WD. A detailed assessment of alterations in bone turnover, calcium homeostasis, and bone density in normal pregnancy. J Bone Miner Res. 2010;15(3):557–63. https://doi.org/10.1359/jbmr.2000.15.3.557.

9. Cross NA, Hillman LS, Allen SH, Krause GF, Vieira NE. Calcium homeostasis and bone metabolism during pregnancy, lactation, and postweaning: a longitudinal study. Am J Clin Nutr. 1995;61(3):514–23. https://doi.org/10.1093/ajcn/61.3.514.

10. Kovacs CS. Maternal mineral and bone metabolism during pregnancy, lactation, and post-weaning recovery. Physiol Rev. 2016;96(2):449–547. https://doi.org/10.1152/physrev.00027.2015.

11. Seely EW, Brown EM, Demaggio DM, Weldon DK, Graves SW. A prospective study of calciotropic hormones in pregnancy and post-partum: reciprocal changes in serum intact parathyroid hormone and 1,25-dihydroxyvitamin D. Am J Obstet Gynecol. 1997;176(1):214–7. https://doi.org/10.1016/s0002-9378(97)80039-7.

12. Ritchie LD, Fung EB, Halloran BP, Turnlund JR, Loan MD, Cann CE, King JC. A longitudinal study of calcium homeostasis during human pregnancy and lactation and after resumption of menses. Am J Clin Nutr. 1998;67(4):693–701. https://doi.org/10.1093/ajcn/67.4.693.

13. Mitchell DM, Regan S, Cooley MR, Lauter KB, Vrla MC, Becker CB, et al. Long-term follow-up of patients with hypoparathyroidism. J Clin Endocrinol Metabol. 2012;97(12):4507–14. https://doi.org/10.1210/jc.2012-1808.

14. Yadav S, Yadav YS, Goel MM, Singh U, Natu SM, Negi MP. Calcitonin gene- and parathyroid hormone-related peptides in normotensive and preeclamptic pregnancies: a nested case–

control study. Arch Gynecol Obstet. 2014;290(5):897–903. https://doi.org/10.1007/s00404-014-3303-8.

15. Eller-Vainicher C, Ossola MW, Beck-Peccoz P, Chiodini I. PTHrP-associated hypercalcemia of pregnancy resolved after delivery: a case report. Eur J Endocrinol. 2012;166(4):753–6. https://doi.org/10.1530/eje-11-1050.

16. Jackson IT, Saleh J, Heerden JA. Gigantic mammary hyperplasia in pregnancy associated with pseudohyperparathyroidism. Plast Reconstr Surg. 1989;84(5):806–10. https://doi.org/10.1097/00006534-198911000-00016.

17. Graham WP, Gordan GS, Loken HF, Blum A, Halden A. Effect of pregnancy and of the menstrual cycle on hypoparathyroidism. J Clin Endocrinol Metab. 1964;24(6):512–6. https://doi.org/10.1210/jcem-24-6-512.

18. Saggese G, Baroncelli G, Bertelloni S, Cipolloni C. Intact parathyroid hormone levels during pregnancy, in healthy term neonates and in hypocalcemic preterm infants. Acta Paediatr. 1991;80(1):36–41. https://doi.org/10.1111/j.1651-2227.1991.tb11726.x.

19. Yamamoto M, Akatsu T, Nagase T, Ogata E. Comparison of hypocalcemic hypercalciuria between patients with idiopathic hypoparathyroidism and those with gain-of-function mutations in the calcium-sensing receptor: is it possible to differentiate the two disorders? J Clin Endocrinol Metabol. 2000;85(12):4583–91. https://doi.org/10.1210/jcem.85.12.7035.

20. Macisaac R, Heath J, Rodda C, Moseley J, Care A, Martin T, Caple I. Role of the fetal parathyroid glands and parathyroid hormone-related protein in the regulation of placental transport of calcium, magnesium and inorganic phosphate. Reprod Fertil Dev. 1991;3(4):447. https://doi.org/10.1071/rd9910447.

21. Trotter M, Hixon BB. Sequential changes in weight, density, and percentage ash weight of human skeletons from an early fetal period through old age. Anat Rec. 1974;179(1):1–18. https://doi.org/10.1002/ar.1091790102.

22. Glass EJ, Barr DG. Transient neonatal hyperparathyroidism secondary to maternal pseudohypoparathyroidism. Arch Dis Child. 1981;56(7):565–8. https://doi.org/10.1136/adc.56.7.565.

23. Loughead J, Mughal Z, Mimouni F, Tsang R, Oestreich A. Spectrum and natural history of congenital hyperparathyroidism secondary to maternal hypocalcemia. Am J Perinatol. 1990;7(04):350–5. https://doi.org/10.1055/s-2007-999521.

24. Stuart C, Aceto T, Kuhn JP, Terplan K. Intrauterine hyperparathyroidism. Am J Dis Child. 1979;133(1):67. https://doi.org/10.1001/archpedi.1979.02130010073013.
25. Vidailhet M, Monin P, Andre M, Suty Y, Marchal C, Vert P. Neonatal hyperparathyroidism secondary to maternal hypoparathyroidism. Archives Francaises De Pediatrie. 1980;37:305–12.
26. Alikasifoglu A, Gonc EN, Yalcin E, Dogru D, Yordam N. Neonatal hyperparathyroidism due to maternal hypoparathyroidism and vitamin D deficiency: a cause of multiple bone fractures. Clin Pediatr. 2005;44(3):267–9. https://doi.org/10.1177/000992280504400312.
27. Shani H, Sivan E, Cassif E, Simchen MJ. Maternal hypercalcemia as a possible cause of unexplained fetal polyhydramnion: a case series. Am J Obstet Gynecol. 2008;199(4):410.e1. https://doi.org/10.1016/j.ajog.2008.06.092.
28. Mestman JH. Parathyroid disorders of pregnancy. Semin Perinatol. 1998;22(6):485–96. https://doi.org/10.1016/s0146-0005(98)80028-1.
29. Bulloch MN, Carroll DG. When one drug affects 2 patients. J Pharm Pract. 2012;25(3):352–67. https://doi.org/10.1177/0897190012442070.
30. Rubin LP, Posillico JT, Anast CS, Brown EM. Circulating levels of biologically active and immunoreactive intact parathyroid hormone in human newborns. Pediatr Res. 1991;29(2):201–7. https://doi.org/10.1203/00006450-199102000-00020.
31. Landing BH, Kamoshita S. Congenital hyperparathyroidism secondary to maternal hypoparathyroidism. J Pediatr. 1970;77(5):842–7. https://doi.org/10.1016/s0022-3476(70)80245-1.

Index

© Springer Nature Switzerland AG 2020
N. E. Cusano (ed.), *Hypoparathyroidism*,
https://doi.org/10.1007/978-3-030-29433-5